A MULTI-AXIAL CLASSIFICATION OF
CHILD PSYCHIATRIC DISORDERS

A Multi-Axial Classification of Child Psychiatric Disorders

An evaluation of a proposal

by

MICHAEL RUTTER, M.D., F.R.C.P., F.R.C.Psych., D.P.M.

Professor of Child Psychiatry, Institute of Psychiatry, London

DAVID SHAFFER, M.B., M.R.C.P., M.R.C.Psych.

Senior Lecturer in Child Psychiatry, Institute of Psychiatry, London

MICHAEL SHEPHERD, D.M., F.R.C.P., F.R.C.Psych., D.P.M.

Professor of Epidemiological Psychiatry, Institute of Psychiatry, London

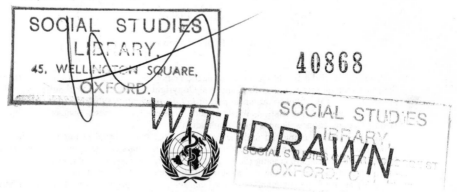

WORLD HEALTH ORGANIZATION

GENEVA

1975

CONTENTS

ACKNOWLEDGEMENTS

The present study was undertaken and conducted with the support of the World Health Organization, as an activity within the framework of the WHO programme on standardization of psychiatric diagnosis, classification, and statistics.

The 22 participants in the study were: Dr P. Barker, Dr L. Bartlet, Dr A. Bentovim, Dr D. Black, Dr A. Bolton, Dr J. Collins, Dr J. Corbett, Dr C. Dennehey, Dr K. Fraser, Dr E. Frommer, Dr P. Graham, Dr M. Heller, Dr L. Hersov, Dr. B. Kirman, Dr I. Kolvin, Dr J. Lindsey, Dr R. Rodriguez, Dr D. Walk, Dr C. Wardle, Dr W. Warren, Dr C. Williams, and Dr S. Wolff. The authors are deeply grateful to these psychiatrists for their help in planning the study, in the extensive work required for its execution, and in the consideration of the implications of the findings. Many of the suggestions in this report about possible improvements in classifications come from them. However, the authors alone are responsible for any shortcomings there may be.

Background

Classification, as a means of ordering information and of grouping phenomena, is basic to all forms of scientific enquiry. This fact was appreciated in medicine over 200 years ago with de Lacroix's classification of diseases (*1*). Since then a number of further needs have been recognized. First, there was the need for uniformity both in the terms used and in the way they are grouped. William Farr emphasized this requirement in the first annual report of the General Register Office of England and Wales in 1839 (*2*), and it was implemented some years later in the International List of Causes of Death. Because the requirement of uniformity necessitated international collaboration and agreement it was natural for the League of Nations and later the World Health Organization (WHO) to be entrusted with the task of preparing approved lists of diseases, together with their classifications. This function has been incorporated in the Constitution of WHO (*3*).

A further need is that classifications should be well designed for the purposes for which they will be used. The International Classification of Diseases (ICD) was originally developed for noting causes of death, and later for providing a single statement of the reasons for admitting inpatients to hospital. The ICD did not correspond well with the kind of statistics required on mental disorders and when, in 1959, Stengel reviewed for WHO the state of psychiatric classification (*4*), he concluded that the ICD had failed to find general acceptance as far as psychiatry was concerned and that major improvements were necessary. Stengel's analysis of the reasons for this failure and his arguments in favour of action were echoed by the first WHO Scientific Group on Mental Health Research, which in 1964 strongly advocated WHO support for the development of a classification of mental disorders internationally acceptable and capable of uniform application.

The Group's recommendation was incorporated in the first of four interrelated programmes that formed the basis of a 10-year research plan formulated by WHO in the mid 1960s (*5, 6*). This programme has been primarily concerned with the standardization of psychiatric diagnosis, classification, and statistics with a view to improving the Ninth Revision of the ICD, which is in preparation. One of its main features has been a series of annual international case-history exercises designed to elucidate the sources of diagnostic variations between representative psychiatrists from many different countries. The method and results of these seminars have served to demonstrate clearly that an experimental approach can not only elucidate many of the sources of disagreement that have long bedevilled progress and communication in this sphere but also indicate how closer agreement can be obtained. In this regard, one of the most important points to emerge has been the need for new schemes of classification based on observation and empirical findings rather than on theoretical models.

It is necessary that classifications should adapt to changing requirements and developing knowledge. When section V of the CID (originally called "Mental, Psychoneurotic and Personality Disorders") was first developed, child psychiatry was in its infancy (7) and no adequate scheme of classification was available. This was still the case in 1960, when the WHO Expert Committee on Mental Health noted both the need for a comprehensive psychiatric classification for childhood and also the lack of such a classification (8). However, that situation has now changed. The third seminar in the WHO programme, which was devoted to child psychiatric disorders, showed that psychiatrists could agree on their classification (9). It was evident that this change would have to be reflected in the Ninth Revision of the ICD but it was equally clear that research would be needed to determine how best this might be done.

The inadequacies of the present ICD (ICD-8)—the Eighth Revision (10)—with respect to mental disorders were underlined in the first seminars in the WHO programme, which was concerned with schizophrenia and related conditions (6). One of the major conclusions reflected the participants' concern regarding the structure of the ICD, and in particular "its inability to provide for the classification of a multifactorial scheme of diagnosis when this is necessary to do justice to a complex clinical situation." Section V (now called "Mental Disorders") contains numerous examples of single rubrics into which heterogeneous types of information have been compressed. Such information may bear on causation (most mental illness is multicausal), premorbid personality, clinical features, or outcome. Logically, some provision should be made for distinguishing between these categories of information by employing some form of "multi-axial" classification for individual conditions. The issue was tackled directly at the third of the WHO seminars, devoted to mental disorders in childhood, which proposed a multi-axial scheme of classification for these disorders (9). In essence, the first axis was intended to cover the clinical psychiatric syndrome, the second to describe the level of intellectual function, and the third to comprise any associated or etiological factors, whether physical or environmental. Subsequently this third axis was split into two (11).

This report describes an attempt by a group of child psychiatrists in the United Kingdom to test and evaluate this scheme.

Multi-axial classification

The desirability of a multi-axial approach to classification has been urged by Essen-Möller in Sweden (12), Helmchen in Germany (36), and Wing in the United Kingdom (13), quite apart from the recommendations made at seminars in the WHO programme. These writers have pointed out that the Eighth Revision of the ICD classifies some psychiatric disorders by symptomatology, some by disease concept, some by etiology, and some by a mixture of all three. This arrangement results in various ambiguities and confusion and it also leads to a loss of important information. Thus, if the case is one of a psychosis associated with brain pathology it is possible to code the type of brain disease but not the type of psychosis. For planning services it would be important to know whether the psychosis took the form of an acute confusional state, dementia, a paranoid state, or a depressive disorder, but this information would be unobtainable from the ICD coding (293). Furthermore, the grouping together of the brain diseases means that differentiation is lost. Thus, Huntington's chorea and multiple sclerosis both receive the same coding (293.4), although they are quite different diseases with different causes, different prognoses, and different mental complications. It has been urged that mental disorders should be classified according to phenomenology on one axis and that etiology should be dealt with on a separate axis.

The need for a multi-axial classification scheme in child psychiatry arose directly out of the case-history exercises in the WHO programme, with respect to patients who showed a psychiatric disorder as well as mental retardation, or a physical condition in association with either (11). Thus, at the third WHO seminar there was a case of a mentally retarded epileptic girl who in addition had a psychiatric disorder. Participants agreed that it was appropriate to code all three elements (psychosis, intellectual retardation, and epilepsy), but in fact most psychiatrists recorded only one, with a fairly even distribution among the three categories chosen for classification. Similarly, at the fifth seminar there was a case of a mentally retarded child with a severe conduct disorder. More than a third of the participants did not record the conduct disorder in their classification, in spite of the fact that they agreed in discussion that it constituted an important part of the diagnosis.

Of course, the ICD does allow the coding of different elements by the use of multiple categories. Thus, it is quite possible to classify the retarded, epileptic, psychotic child by means of ICD-8 categories 311 (mild mental retardation), 345 (epilepsy), and 295.8 (other psychosis, including childhood schizophrenia). However, there are no rules as to how many categories to use and, as the diagnostic exercise clearly showed, psychiatrists varied in the number of codings they employed. Furthermore, when they chose one they differed in their choice. Additionally, in a number of medical centres the rule is to code only one diagnosis per patient.

The net effect is that when the ICD is employed in the usual way it is not possible to obtain a complete list of all patients with mental retardation, or all with a mental disorder, or all with epilepsy. This is because patients with multiple conditions (a common situation) may have only one condition coded. The fact that a condition is not coded may mean that the condition was not present, that it was present but not thought important, or that it was not coded in spite of being thought important. This has serious implications for both planning services and for research. The multi-axial scheme was designed to remedy these deficiencies.

In fact, it is no more than a logical development of a multi-category scheme (such as the ICD) in which modifications have been introduced specifically to meet these difficulties. To ensure adequate coverage of data and to ensure comparability three rules are required: (1) a uniform number of codings must be made, (2) these codings must always refer to the same elements in diagnosis, and (3) they must always occur in the same order. There is an infinite variety of elements that could be included in such a scheme, but for it to be workable in practice there must be a quite restricted number of axes. These need to be chosen on the basis of providing unambiguous information of maximum clinical usefulness in the greatest number of cases. With regard to child psychiatric disorders, the axes that were selected referred to the clinical psychiatric syndrome (neurotic disorders, infantile autism, etc.), to the intellectual level (normal, mildly retarded, etc.), to associated medical conditions (cerebral palsy, asthma, etc.), and to psychological or social factors that might be important in etiology. Most of these items are already in the ICD, so that the multi-axial scheme simply regrouped the categories under four broad headings called "axes". For each axis a "no abnormality" coding is provided and psychiatrists have to make some coding on each of the four axes for every patient. This provision ensures that comparable data on the four elements of diagnosis are coded in the same way and in the same order for all cases, so that systematic data retrieval is a straightforward matter.

This type of classification seemed to overcome the limitations of multi-category schemes such as the ICD and its use was urged in all succeeding seminars in the WHO programme. Nevertheless, whatever its theoretical advantages, it required empirical testing in practice. This testing was one of the main purposes of the present study.

Classification of child psychiatric disorders

The codings for the clinical syndromes in child psychiatry on the first axis of the multi-axial scheme were suggested during the course of the third WHO seminar as the basis for developing an adequate classification. In no sense were they intended to constitute a full coverage of the psychiatric disorders met with in childhood. Rather, they were seen as a skeleton to build on. Ten overall categories were provided, only three of them being subdivided (see Annex 1). It was expected that more subdivisions would be added later in the light of further experience and testing (9).

Aims and objectives

The multi-axial scheme for classifying child psychiatric disorders was therefore new in two respects—the provision of categories specifically for children's disorders and the provision of a multi-axial framework. Both elements needed to be systematically evaluated.

With any model of classification there are a series of criteria which must be applied in order to assess its value. These may be summarized as follows:

1. Reliability

Any scheme that is to be useful must be reliable in the sense that different people will use the system to produce the same codings for the same patients, and that any rater will code the same way when confronted with the same material on different occasions. The case-history exercise developed during the seminars (6) has proved to be a valuable method of testing reliability.

Unreliability, when it exists, may arise from several different sources and in the evaluation of any new classification model, the identification of the sources of unreliability will be an important point of the study. In particular, it is necessary to differentiate unreliability that stems from limitation in psychiatric knowledge or in the experience of psychiatrists from unreliability that is inherent in the classification scheme itself. Some measure of the former may be obtained from the case-history exercise by examining inter-psychiatrist agreement with regard to diagnostic formulations, rating of symptomatology, treatment recommendations, and prognosis.

Homogeneity in the training experience and in the conceptional framework of psychiatrists using a classification is likely to increase the extent to which they agree with one another in coding diagnosis. However, an international classification must be applicable and reliable in spite of wide differences in theoretical orientation. Accordingly, participants in the study were deliberately chosen so as to be varied in outlook. Even so, they were probably more similar in outlook than psychiatrists from different countries, so that testing in other parts of the world and with respect to patients from differing cultures is still required. These sources of unreliability may be minimized by ensuring familiarity with a comprehensive glossary. However, only a partial pilot version of a glossary was available for the present study.

A further issue related to reliability is the spread of diagnoses. Where only a very limited range of codings is used, reliability will be artificially high. High reliability in coding must not be achieved at the expense of failure to discriminate between different psychiatric conditions. This means that a classification's powers of differentiation between various disorders must be assessed.

Finally, there will be a particular interest in situations where psychiatrists agree on their diagnostic formulation of a case but nevertheless still disagree on their coding of this diagnosis in the classification scheme. This type of unreliability results directly from defects in the scheme itself.

2. Information demands

In order for a classification to be generally serviceable it is necessary to determine what sort and what amount of information is required to classify disorders according to the scheme. In short, can classification be made on the basis of a brief interview, does it need a hospital-type assessment, or must it await extensive investigations or follow-up findings? Can diagnosis be made on a present mental state examination or does it require historical information, including findings on family history or environmental influences? These issues can be investigated experimentally, as done by Kendell (14), or they can be assessed by means of field trials, as done in the present study.

3. Use in routine practice

Developing out of the question of information demands is the need for a classification to be applicable to the conditions existing in ordinary clinical practice. It must be acceptable to clinicians, and the instructions on its use must be clear, simple, and unambiguous. For this purpose a new element in methodology was provided by introducing the multi-axial classification in the setting of routine clinical practice (15). In this way it was hoped to assess the acceptability and feasibility of the scheme in ordinary psychiatric work, both outpatient and inpatient, and to determine how often the various diagnostic categories were used.

4. Validity

For the categories used in any classification to have any meaning it must be shown that they differ in some respect. It is not enough that tradition or theory separate two conditions; it is also essential that in fact they differ in terms of etiology, symptomatology, course, response to treatment, or some other variable (16). It should be a basic principle that differentiations between categories may only be retained in a classification if they can be shown empirically to have some demonstrable value. In the present study it was possible to examine these issues in only a very limited way. However, information was systematically sought on the symptoms, family background, treatment, and course of the disorder over one year in order to make a start on this aspect of evaluation.

5. Comparisons with other models

It is not enough to show that a new system of classification is useful. It is also necessary to show that it is superior to previous models in certain specific respects. Because the ICD is the generally accepted scheme for classifying psychiatric disorders it was evident that the new scheme should be compared directly with it in order to assess its advantages and disadvantages.

6. Statistical considerations

Because the data deriving from any classification will be used to produce a variety of statistics, an essential element in testing is the production of statistical tables showing how the data produced by a new model of classification may be presented. In this connexion, the criteria to be applied will include the range of questions to which it can be applied, the simplicity of presentation, the comprehensibility of statistical tables based on the new model of classification, the ease of information storage and retrieval, and the feasibility of computer programming. These elements could most easily be tested in the clinical study using the classification in ordinary clinical practice.

Research design and methodology

Classification schemes

The two schemes of classification to be compared were the Eighth Revision of the International Classification of Diseases (ICD-8) and the multi-axial system (MAS) of classification of child psychiatric disorders suggested at the WHO seminar held in Paris in 1967 (9) and further developed by the seminar on mental retardation held in Washington, DC, in 1969 (11)

In effect, the comparison involves two quite different types of question. The first issue is how well the two classifications (ICD-8 and MAS) provide for the coding of child psychiatric disorders. In this connexion, it should be appreciated that ICD-8 was developed at a time when there was little agreement concerning classification in child psychiatry. Accordingly, the limitations of ICD-8 reflect the limitations of psychiatric knowledge at the time it was planned. This study was possible because of advances in child psychiatry, and the point of this comparison was to determine what provision for child psychiatric disorders might be introduced into the next edition of the ICD, now in preparation.

The second issue is whether a multi-axial system of classification, with the coding structure implicit in such a system, has advantages over a multi-category system without that structure. Here the point is not the content or range of the categories but rather the way in which the system is organized and the nature of the coding instructions on its use. As already noted, although the ICD is not ordinarily used as a multi-axial system, with quite minor modifications it could be ordered in that way. In short, the basic question being asked in this part of the study was what, if any, gains would follow from giving the ICD a multi-axial structure.

Participants were given the British glossary (17)[a] for section V of ICD-8, together with a list of the main codings in other sections of the ICD. They were also provided with the paper describing the rationale of the MAS and with a brief provisional glossary listing and describing the psychiatric syndromes included (9). The MAS consisted of four axes, each made up of a list of categories and codings (see Annex 1). The axes were: (a) child psychiatric syndrome, (b) level of intellectual functioning, (c) associated or etiological biological influences, and (d) associated or etiological psychosocial influences. For each patient, participants had to make one coding only on each axis.

The axis of psychiatric syndromes consisted of a provisional list of the main disorders met with in child psychiatry. Adult conditions were not included, but

---

[a] No WHO glossary was available at the time of the study.

the aim of the third WHO seminar was that, after appropriate testing and revision, the children's disorders should then be incorporated into section V of the ICD.

The Paris and Washington seminars did not provide glossaries or full listings for the other three axes, so that schemes had to be developed for the purposes of the study. The intellectual axis followed the subdivision and instructions suggested at the seminars, but no glossary was drawn up. The biological influence axis consisted simply of a summary (with minor modification) of the ICD scheme for classifying medical conditions other than psychiatric disorders. Because of the special importance of neurological conditions in psychiatry, greater weight was given to these in devising the summary classification.

No similar model was available for the classification of psychosocial factors, so that an *ad hoc* scheme had to be produced. Following preliminary discussions with the psychiatrists participating in the study, a short list of categories was made; this constituted the psychosocial axis. No glossaries were provided for axes other than the first.

Selection of participants

The report of the Paris seminar was discussed and an outline of the proposed study was given at a general meeting of the Royal Medico-Psychological Association (now the Royal College of Psychiatrists), London. Consultant psychiatrists were invited to participate and 22 agreed to do so, including people working in various settings: paediatric hospitals, undergraduate teaching hospitals, child guidance clinics, mental retardation units, academic centres, and other specialized and general clinics. Their theoretical orientation was quite varied and there were both psychoanalytically and "organically" oriented psychiatrists. However, most adopted an eclectic approach.

Organization of the study

All participants met beforehand to plan the investigation and to discuss methods and objectives, in order to ensure uniformity of procedure in carrying out the study. After completion of each of the two studies and analysis of their data, an all-day meeting was held with the participants to discuss the findings and to arrive at agreed recommendations. The conclusions of this report embody the results of the discussions.

Reliability study

The reliability study was based on the agreement/disagreement between participants on their diagnostic coding of 17 case histories distributed by post (see Annex 2). These covered a wide range of problems, both straightforward and complex or atypical, in children who had been followed for at least two years and for whom there was good documentation. The histories were between 4000 and 5000 words in length and were prepared in two parts. The second was sent to participants only after diagnostic codings had been made on the first part and the standard forms returned. The first part provided the information available at the time of initial assessment on presenting symptoms with details of manner of onset, duration, course and precipitants; personal history and schooling; family history and family relationships; mental state examination, psychological testing, and clinical investigations carried out at the time of initial assessment. The second part described the treatment given, the child's response, and his state at the time of follow-up.

Participants were asked to rate on a standard form a number of listed symptoms, to note their recommendations on treatment, and to assess prognosis with respect to both symptomatology and social adjustment a year after the initial attendance. They were requested to provide a diagnostic formulation in their own words and to select one or more diagnostic codings from the ICD and also one for each axis on the multi-axial system (MAS). Comments were asked for on any difficulties experienced in classifying cases on either system.

After ratings on the first part had been returned, the second part of the summary (giving follow-up data) was sent to the participants, who were invited to amend their diagnosis in the light of the further information if they so wished.

Clinical study

The reliability study was designed to provide information on how well psychiatrists could agree on classification when given standard information. However, it could not provide data on how well any classification scheme works in the conditions of ordinary clinical practice and inevitably only a limited range of disorders could be covered by 17 case-histories. To meet both of these needs, each participant was asked to complete similar forms (on diagnosis, symptomatology, etc.) on 10–15 consecutive new referrals to their own clinics. In order to determine whether adequate information for coding would ordinarily be available in outpatient practice, most cases were outpatients, but some inpatients were also included. Information on 255 cases was provided in this way. Systematic follow-up at 6 months and 12 months was requested and forms were completed on 165 children at 6 months and 177 at 12 months. Follow-up information at one or other time was available for 212 children.

Reliability of diagnostic coding on psychiatric syndrome (first axis of MAS)

In order to compare the merits and demerits of the Eighth Edition of the ICD with those of the MAS, the reliability findings on each are presented together. The overall figures of agreement were virtually identical for the two schemes, averaging 67%.[a] However, the strengths and weaknesses of each lay in different directions, as can readily be seen when cases are grouped according to diagnostic similarity. In all tables, agreement is expressed as the percentage of psychiatrists who have used the code employed by the greatest number of participants in diagnosing a given case.

Neurotic disorders (cases 2, 3, and 8)

There were 3 cases with a reasonably well defined neurotic disorder—a 13-year-old boy with a hysterical paralysis of one leg, a 6-year-old boy with a disabling dog phobia, and a 10-year-old girl with numerous anxieties and school refusal. On both the ICD and the MAS there was no difficulty in identifying all 3 cases as some form of neurotic disorder and on both schemes there was a high level of inter-rater agreement. However, the ICD gave more information concerning the type of neurotic disorder.

TABLE 1
INTER-RATER AGREEMENT ON FIRST AXIS AND ICD CODINGS (CASES 2, 3, AND 8)

Case No.	Most common code		Second most common code		Description of case
	Code	Used by (%)	Code	Used by (%)	
Inter-rater agreement on first axis coding					
2	4	86	8.5	9	Hysterical paralysis
3	4	95	8.5	5	Dog phobia
8	4	91	1	9	School refusal
Inter-rater agreement on ICD coding					
2	300.1	72	300.0	14	Hysterical paralysis
3	300.2	100	—	—	Dog phobia
8	300.0	54	300.2	36	School refusal

On the MAS the great majority of participants coded 4 (neurotic disorder) for all three cases. On the ICD nearly everyone used one of the 300 codes (for neurosis). On the first case there was quite good agreement on the more

[a]On both schemes agreement was calculated on the basis of coding subdivisions where these were available. On the first axis of the MAS, 13 of the available 24 codes were used on at least 5 occasions and on the ICD, 15 of the 124 available codes were used at least 5 times.

specific fourth digit coding of 300.1 (hysterical neurosis), on the second everyone coded 300.2 (phobic neurosis), but on the third there was a split between 300.0 (anxiety neurosis) and 300.2 (phobic neurosis).

As these fourth-digit distinctions were made with some reliability it would seem desirable also to include this differentiation in the MAS by a subdivision of code 4.

Depressive disorder (case 5)

Case 5 (a socially withdrawn boy presenting with depression, derealization, retardation, and insomnia) gave rise to some difficulties with both systems of classification. Nearly all the participants considered him to have a depressive disorder; there was a majority coding of 4 (neurotic disorder) on the MAS and a majority coding of 300.4 (depressive neurosis) on the ICD. However, the severity of the depression and its association with derealization and retardation led a significant minority to make a psychotic coding.

TABLE 2
INTER-RATER AGREEMENT ON FIRST AXIS AND ICD CODINGS (CASE 5)

	Most common code		Second most common code		
	Code	Used by (%)*	Code	Used by (%)	Description of case
Multi-axial code	4	54	5.4	23	Depression, derealization, retardation, and
ICD code	300.4	63	296	18	social withdrawal

Again, the MAS failed to provide adequate differentiation as depression (unless psychotic) had to be grouped with all other neurotic disorders. Participants pointed to the need for a specific coding for depression. The difficulty with the ICD was the problem, common to both child and adult psychiatry, of the uncertain and poorly defined differentiations between manic-depressive psychosis, reactive depressive psychosis, and depressive neurosis. Many participants considered that these were not the appropriate distinctions to be made within the general category of depression. The facts that are required to decide how depressive disorders can be best subdivided are not yet available and clearly this is an area requiring further research.

Mild emotional disorders in young children (cases 7 and 15)

Cases 7 (a 6-year-old girl with tearfulness after a long separation from her mother) and 15 (a 3½-year-old girl with tantrums apparently related to stresses associated with a retarded brother) were both examples of mild emotional disorders in young children. In both cases the majority coding on the ICD was 308 (behaviour disorders of childhood), a very general coding that gave no useful information about either the type or the severity of the disorder. For case 7 the second most frequent coding was 300.4 (depressive neurosis), which describes the type of disorder, and for case 15 the second most frequent coding was 307 (transient situational disturbance), which describes the severity. On the MAS the majority coding for the first case was 4 (neurotic disorder), with 1

TABLE 3
INTER-RATER AGREEMENT ON 1ST AXIS AND ICD CODINGS (CASES 7 AND 15)

Case No.	Most common code		Second most common code		Description of case
	Code	Used by (%)	Code	Used by (%)	
7: 1st axis code	4	54	1	36	Tearfulness in a 6-year-
ICD code	308	45	300.4	45	old girl
15: 1st axis code	1	59	4	36	Tantrums and
					babyishness in a 3-year-
ICD code	308	63	307	27	old girl

(adaptation reaction) as the second most frequent coding. For the second case the order was reversed, with adaptation reaction as the majority coding.

The MAS coding gave more precise information in both cases and was therefore the more satisfactory system. Because adaptation reaction was defined in terms of severity rather than of duration it proved to be a more suitable coding than the comparable ICD coding 307 (transient situational disturbance). Nevertheless, on both systems it was impossible to specify the type of disorder if a coding based mainly on severity was made. Further subdivision of both adaptation reaction (on the MAS) and transient situational disturbance (on the ICD) was therefore indicated.

Conduct disorders (cases 1, 9, 6, and 17)

Cases 1, 9, 6, and 17 received different majority diagnoses on the MAS but all were given a majority coding of 308 on the ICD.

On case 1 (an adolescent who showed severely defiant and violent behaviour at home but who posed no problems at school) the choice differed between MAS codings 4 (neurotic disorder) and 3 (conduct disorder) and there was general agreement between participants on the need for a coding that could be used for mixed emotional and conduct disorders. Total agreement on the ICD coding of 308 (behaviour disorder of childhood) was obtained at the expense of using a code that gives no information about the characteristics of the disorder.

Case 9 was the rather complicated one of a solitary and suspicious boy who bullied other children and who developed paranoid ideas during the follow-up period. On the MAS there was a majority coding of 6 (personality disorder), with 4 (neurotic disorder) being the second most frequent coding. On the ICD the majority coding was again 308, with 301.0 (paranoid personality) as the second most frequent coding. Altogether, 6 of the 301 codes were used, indicating the great unreliability of distinctions between different types of personality disorder. This case also illustrates the difficulty with both systems of classification of deciding when a long-standing behavioural disturbance should be regarded as a personality disorder.

Case 6 (a mentally retarded 6-year-old with a long history of over-activity, short attention span, and aggression) gave rise to a high measure of agreement on the MAS coding 2.1 (hyperkinetic disorder). There is no equivalent coding on the ICD and most participants settled for the general coding of 308. The next most frequent ICD coding was 311.4 (mental retardation), which refers to the intellectual level rather than to the type of psychiatric disorder. This case illustrates both the non-specificity of the ICD 308 coding and also the problem with the ICD of deciding whether to code on the basis of the psychiatric disorder, the intellectual level, or both.

Case 17 (persistent stealing in an adolescent boy) was coded 3 (conduct disorder) on the MAS by most of the participants, with 6 (personality disorder) as the second most frequent coding. The ICD codings were similar, with 308 being used most often, followed by 301.7 (antisocial personality). This case again demonstrates the non-specificity of 308 but also shows the difficulty with any classification system of deciding between long-standing illness and a personality disorder.

Taken as a group these cases demonstrated the superiority of the MAS listing of children's disorders in differentiating between a conduct disorder, a personality disorder, and the hyperkinetic syndrome. Neither system, however, was able to distinguish the case of a mixed emotional and conduct disorder.

TABLE 4
INTER-RATER AGREEMENT ON FIRST AXIS AND ICD CODINGS (CASES 1, 9, 6, AND 17)

	Most common code		Second most common code		
Case No.	Code	Used by (%)	Code	Used by (%)	Description of case
Inter-rater agreement on first axis coding					
1	4	50	3	32	Adolescent aggression at home, no problems at school.
9	6	59	4	18	Solitary, suspicious bully. Paranoid ideas.
6	2.1	81	3	9	Overactivity, poor concentration, aggression.
17	3	63	6	25	Stealing and truancy.
Inter-rater agreement on ICD coding					
1	308	100	—	—	Adolescent aggression at home, no problems at school.
9	308	59	301.0	18	Solitary, suspicious bully. Paranoid ideas.
6	308	59	311.4	31	Overactivity, poor concentration, aggression.
17	308	63	301.7	56	Stealing and truancy.

Cases with either organic conditions or intellectual retardation in addition to psychiatric disorder (cases 10, 11, and 12)

All participants coded case 10 (a mentally retarded girl with mild behavioural and emotional disturbance) as mental retardation on the ICD, but there was some disagreement about its severity. On the MAS first axis half the participants coded 9 (manifestation of mental subnormality alone) and one-third 4 (neurotic disorder). This discrepancy shows that the clinical problem of deciding how much disturbance is to be expected on the basis of intellectual impairment alone was more difficult than any coding problem as such.

Case 11 (an 8-year-old girl with progressive dementia) was coded 8.2 on the MAS by most participants but a few coded 8.1 (acute confusional state). The intellectual impairment was described on the second axis and the underlying neurological disorder on the third axis. It is in this sort of case with a psychiatric disorder, intellectual impairment, and a medical condition that the MAS most clearly showed its superiority. On the ICD nearly half coded 323 (encephalitis) but a quarter coded 293 (psychosis with intracranial infection), which illustrates the dilemma of whether to code the psychiatric syndrome or the neurological condition.

Case 12 was an unusually complicated disorder involving long-standing behavioural disturbance in an epileptic boy who presented with petit mal status. It was not adequately classified on either system. There was wide disagreement on the MAS coding, a quarter of the participants coding 8.1 (confusional disorder), a fifth 3 (conduct disorder), and another fifth 6 (personality disorder). Agreement was somewhat better on the ICD but no more satisfactory, 50% of the participants making more than one diagnosis. Half coded 309 (non-psychotic organic disorder), which took note of the organic element but did not specify the type of disorder, and half coded the epilepsy separately. Another third coded 308 (behaviour disorder of childhood), which was even more non-specific, and a quarter coded 310 (mental retardation). It is apparent that exceptionally complex cases are poorly covered by both classification systems.

TABLE 5
INTER-RATER AGREEMENT ON FIRST AXIS AND ICD CODINGS (CASES 10, 11, AND 12)

Case No.	Most common code		Second most common code		Description of case
	Code	Used by (%)	Code	Used by (%)	
10: 1st axis code	9	50	4	33	Mentally retarded girl with minor
ICD code	311	77	313	23	behavioural disturbance
11: 1st axis code	8.2	75	8.1	10	Progressive dementia
ICD code	323	48	293	24	
12: 1st axis code	8.1	27	3	18	Aggression, wandering, and dream
ICD code	309	50	345	45	states in an epileptic boy

Psychosis (cases 13 and 14)

Cases 13 and 14 were both examples of psychotic disorders. There was almost unanimous agreement in coding case 14 (a deluded and hallucinated 14-year-old) as schizophrenic on both systems of classification. Case 13 (a 13-year-old boy with infantile autism that had arisen on the basis of congenital syphilis) was coded on the ICD as 090 (congenital syphilis) by two-thirds of participants and 292 (psychosis associated with intracranial infection) by nearly half, which again reflects the dilemma of which aspect of the case to code. Three-quarters of the participants used more than one coding. On the MAS most participants coded 5.1 (infantile psychosis), a code not available on the ICD, which provides no specific coding for this type of psychosis.

TABLE 6
INTER-RATER AGREEMENT ON FIRST AXIS AND ICD CODINGS (CASES 13 AND 14)

Case No.	Most common code		Second most common code		Description of case
	Code	Used by (%)	Code	Used by (%)	
13: 1st axis code	5.1	68	5.4	9	Infantile autism in a boy with
ICD code	090	69	292	45	congenital syphilis
14: 1st axis code	5.3	100	—,	—	Schizophrenia in an adolescent
ICD code	295	95	297	5	

Miscellaneous disorders (cases 4 and 16)

The case of cross-dressing in an adolescent boy (case 4) was almost unanimously coded 302 (sexual deviation) on the ICD. There was good agreement on a coding of 6 (personality disorder) on the MAS, but this was unsatisfactory in that it failed to indicate the specifically sexual nature of the disorder. Case 16, an encopretic girl, was coded 2.6 on the MAS, and 306.1 on the ICD by most participants, both codes being reserved for cases of encopresis.

TABLE 7
INTER-RATER AGREEMENT ON FIRST AXIS AND ICD CODINGS (CASES 4 AND 16)

	Most common code		Second most common code		
Case No.	Code	Used by (%)	Code	Used by (%)	Description of case
4: 1st axis code	6	63	8.5	23	Cross-dressing in a 15-year-old
ICD code	302	95	301.6	9	boy
16: 1st axis code	2.6	63	4	18	Encopresis in an 11-year-old girl
ICD code	306.1	77	308	27	

In general, therefore, the findings on diagnostic coding of psychiatric disorder showed a similar level of inter-rater reliability for both systems. Reliability of coding was moderately good for most cases but it fell to low levels on some of the very complicated cases. The MAS was better suited to cases where a psychiatric disorder was associated with a neurological condition and it allowed more precise coding of cases of conduct disorder, hyperkinetic disorder, and infantile psychosis. The ICD permitted better differentiation among the neuroses and personality disorders and a more precise coding for depression and sexual deviation.

Reliability of coding on intellectual level (second axis of the MAS)

In 9 of the 17 cases there was 100% agreement on a coding of normal intelligence. In a further 2 cases there was better than 90% agreement on the same coding. There was total agreement on a coding of mental retardation in one case and at least 90% agreement in 2 further cases. In one case there was 86% agreement on a mental retardation coding, in another 64% agreement. In one case 77% coded normal intelligence and 23% coded "not known". There was less agreement on the degree of intellectual impairment.

TABLE 8
INTER-RATER AGREEMENT ON SECOND AXIS CODING

	Most common coding		Second most common coding	
Case No.	Code	Used by (%)	Code	Used by (%)
1	0	100	—	
2	0	100	—	
3	0	100	—	
4	0	91	1	9
5	0	100	—	
6	1	68	2	18
7	0	95	1	5
8	0	100	—	
9	0	100	—	
10	2	68	3	32
11	4	35	5	26
12	1	63	2	27
13	1	41	0	36
14	0	77	9	23
15	0	100	—	
16	0	100	—	
17	0	100	—	

Much the most frequent cause of disagreement over the coding of intellectual impairment was the presence of conflicting IQ scores on either different tests or different occasions. This situation arose particularly in cases where there was a marked difference between the verbal and performance scores on the Wechsler scales. Case 11 gave rise to different difficulties in that the girl was rapidly deteriorating and participants were uncertain about which stage in the disease process should be used to rate intellectual level.

Reliability of coding on biological factors (third axis of the MAS)

There were too few cases involving a medical condition to warrant systematic study of inter-rater agreement on the third axis. However, even from the few cases included it was evident that there were problems. With case 11 (a girl with subacute sclerosing leucoencephalitis) there was considerable variation on the third axis coding when it had to be made on the first part of the case history at a time when the cause of her dementia was not certainly known. Two-fifths (38%) of the participants coded 8.4 (progressive cerebral atrophy of unknown etiology) and one-third 1.5 (encephalopathies associated with infection). The alternative coding (1.5) was "correct" in that it took account of the specific etiology but its use shows that when etiology is uncertain the same condition may be coded in quite different sections of the classification. As the third axis is simply a summary of ICD codings, this criticism applies to the ICD as a whole. This wide difference in the coding arises because some ICD codings are made on the basis of specific etiological factors and some on the basis of phenomenology.

A similar problem arose with case 13, the boy with congenital syphilis, where two-thirds of the participants (67%) coded 1.0 (spirochaetal disease of the CNS) but 13% coded 0.1 (infective aparasitic non-neurological condition). This particular difficulty would not have arisen in the full ICD, where the fuller specification of codings (congenital syphilis of all types share one 3-digit coding) makes it clearer than did the third axis which coding should be made. With case 12 (the boy with petit mal status) half the participants coded 8.2 (epilepsy), but 13% coded 8.5 (other chronic neurological syndromes) because of the uncertainty as to whether 8.2 should include dream states due to petit mal status. Here too, the greater specificity of the full ICD would have avoided this particular difficulty.

However, use of the ICD could not avoid the difficulties in case 6, the hyperkinetic boy with clumsiness, speech delay, and a history of a threatened miscarriage during the pregnancy. On the third axis, a quarter (27%) of the participants coded 8.3 (chronic encephalopathy of an unspecified nature), a quarter coded 0.0 (no abnormality), and a quarter coded one of the "7" codes (specific developmental disorder). This divergence demonstrates the coding difficulty when there is a mixture of non-specific neurological abnormalities of unknown etiology that does not constitute a known syndrome. Neither the ICD nor the MAS provides a satisfactory coding solution in these circumstances.

Reliability of coding on psychosocial factors (fourth axis of the MAS)

The fourth axis coding proved almost totally unsatisfactory, because of both low reliability and lack of discrimination. The overall level of agreement of coding was only 48% and 11 of the 17 cases all received the same majority coding—1 (disorder of intrafamilial relationships; hostility, rejection, lack of warmth, etc.). In two cases there was a high level of agreement (77% and 100%) on the presence of a normal psychosocial situation but one of these was a case of mental retardation and the other was the purely organic case of sub-acute sclereosing leucoencephalitis. While psychiatrists are agreed on the importance of noting psychosocial influences in any diagnostic formulation, the present scheme for coding such factors was clearly inadequate.

TABLE 9
INTER-RATER AGREEMENT ON FOURTH AXIS CODING

Case No.	Most common coding		Second most common coding	
	Code	Used by (%)	Code	Used by (%)
1	1	45	3	40
2	1	63	2	19
3	1	54	7	23
4	1	40	0	27
5	1	68	2	13
6	1	54	0	27
7	6	36	5	32
8	2	36	1	32
9	1	40	3	27
10	0	77	2	9
11	0	100	—	—
12	1	63	0	27
13	1	54	2	18
14	1	63	5	9
15	1	45	9	27
16	2	50	1	41
17	3	25	5	25

Multiple coding

There were 5 cases in which the majority of participants noted mental retardation on the second axis of the MAS (case 6—86%, case 10—100%, case 11—90%, case 12—95%, and case 13—55%). This aspect of the diagnosis was recorded much less often on the ICD. In case 6 it was noted by 49% of the participants, in case 10 by 100%, in case 11 by 5%, in case 12 by 33%, and in case 13 by 27%. The only case in which all the participants made a coding of mental retardation on the ICD was one where retardation was the main reason for referral. When some kind of behavioural disturbance in a mentally retarded child led to referral, participants varied widely on whether they considered that the retardation should receive an ICD coding. It may be concluded that when cases involved both a clinical psychiatric disorder and mental retardation the MAS provided much more consistent and reliable codings.

The same applied to the few cases with an associated medical condition. With case 12, the epilepsy was noted by means of a combination code by 50% of the participants and by means of a separate coding (345) by 45%. With case 13, the congenital syphilis received a separate coding from 68% of the participants. Some also made a combination code, but others failed to record the congenital syphilis by any coding.

Agreement on symptomatology, treatment, and prognosis

To ascertain the source of unreliability in cases where agreement on diagnostic coding proved to be low, it was necessary to determine as accurately as possible to what extent the problems derived from the diagnostic coding *per se* or from lack of agreement on symptomatology, treatment, prognosis, and other aspects of the clinical assessment. On each of the case histories, the participants were asked to make a coding for each of these areas. Naturally, the codings had to be made on the basis of a written description of the case and not on the participants' own clinical examination.

Symptomatology

There was a moderate level of agreement on symptomatology, as shown in Table 10, which is based on the first 16 cases (symptoms were not coded on case 17). The table shows agreement on the presence or absence of a recorded symptom regardless of severity. As the symptoms varied greatly in frequency, agreement (in terms of 60% or greater) is given separately for the absence of a symptom and for its presence.

TABLE 10
INTER-RATER AGREEMENT ON SYMPTOMS

	Level of agreement					
	60% or better agreement on absence of symptom		41–59% agreement (i.e., near chance range)		60% or better agreement on presence of symptom	
Symptom	No. of cases	(%)	No. of cases	(%)	No. of cases	(%)
Emotional disturbance	0	0	1	6	15	93
Obsessions	9	56	3	19	4	25
Stereotypies	12	75	3	19	1	6
Autism	14	87	1	6	1	6
Disturbed family relationships	1	6	1	6	14	87
Disturbed peer relationships	3	19	2	12	11	68
Antisocial behaviour	4	25	6	37	6	37
Hyperkinesis	13	81	1	6	2	12
Educational retardation	6	37	3	19	7	44

Some symptoms (such as emotional disturbance, disturbed family relationships, and disturbed peer relationships) were recorded in such a high proportion of cases that they were of little discriminative value. Others (such as stereotypies, autism, and hyperkinesis) occurred in only a few cases but were of some diagnostic importance when they were present. The least satisfactory agreement was on antisocial behaviour, where a third of cases showed agreement in the near-chance range (41–59%). Participants evidently found it difficult both to decide which forms of behaviour should be included under this heading and to avoid the influence of value judgements.

Some of this unreliability may have stemmed from forcing codings into an arbitrary "present" or "absent" categorization. However, when correlations based on the 4-point scale of severity of symptoms were calculated instead, the pattern of findings was broadly similar. The average product/moment correlation between participants was moderate for most symptoms (e.g., educational retardation—0.64, disturbed peer relationships—0.56, obsessions—0.59) but that for antisocial behaviour was quite low—0.26.

Treatment

There was a generally high level of agreement on treatment (although it remains uncertain how far this was affected by the way the case was described in the case history). The most commonly advocated treatment (6 cases) was a combination of psychotherapy with the child and casework with the parents. Drugs were advocated by most participants in cases of depression, hyperkinetic syndrome, epilepsy, autism, and schizophrenia. Inpatient treatment was most often recommended for the organic and psychotic cases (encephalitis, petit mal status, autism, and schizophrenia), but it was also advised by most participants for the cases of depression and the hyperkinetic syndrome. Behaviour modification treatments were suggested for the case of dog phobia by nearly everyone, and supportive treatment was recommended by the majority of participants for the retarded girl and for the 3-year-old with tantrums.

TABLE 11
INTER-RATER AGREEMENT ON TREATMENT

Case	Most common coding		Second most common coding	
	Code	Used by (%)	Code	Used by (%)
1	Casework with parents	100	Psychotherapy for child	95
2	Casework with parents	90	Psychotherapy for child	90
3	Behaviour modification	86	Supportive treatment	77
4	Psychotherapy for child	86	Casework with parents	81
5	Drugs	95	Inpatient treatment	90
6	Drugs	100	Inpatient treatment	95
7	Casework with parents	81	Psychotherapy for child	50
8	Psychotherapy for child	95	Casework with parents	95
9	Casework with parents	90	Psychotherapy for child	81
10	Supportive treatment	90	Drugs	23
11	Inpatient treatment	81	Drugs	36
12	Drugs	90	Inpatient treatment	63
13	Drugs	86	Inpatient treatment	77
14	Drugs	100	Inpatient treatment	100
15	Supportive treatment	81	Casework with parents	72
16	Casework with parents	77	Inpatient treatment	77

Prognosis

In general there was reasonably good agreement on prognosis, the average product/moment correlation, in the event of the case receiving optimal treatment, being 0.64 on symptoms 1 year later and 0.69 on social adjustment. The agreement on prognosis, assuming the treatment likely to be available, was lower (0.44 for symptoms and 0.57 for social adjustment).

Prognostic assessments also differentiated well between cases, as shown in Table 12. A favourable prognosis was given for both symptoms and social adjustment with respect to cases 3 (dog phobia), 7 (tearfulness in a 6-year-old), 8 (school refusal), 15 (tantrums in a 3-year-old), and 16 (encopresis). Unfavourable prognoses on both symptoms and social adjustment were given for

TABLE 12
PROGNOSIS SCORES,[a] ASSUMING OPTIMAL TREATMENT

Case No.	Symptoms	Social adjustment
3	11	8
7	20	14
8	15	22
15	6	20
16	21	20
1	29	23
2	24	30
4	35	12
5	28	39
10	34	35
17	32	30
6	53	54
9	46	45
11	60	63
12	47	48
13	57	57
14	53	58

[a] A low score indicates a good prognosis.

cases 6 (hyperkinetic syndrome), 9 (solitary, suspicious bully), 11 (encephalitis), 12 (epileptic with a conduct disorder), 13 (autism), and 14 (schizophrenia).

It may be concluded that there was a fairly satisfactory level of agreement between clinicians in their judgements on symptomatology, treatment, and prognosis but that the inter-observer variation was sufficient to account for a good deal of the unreliability in diagnostic coding.

Change of diagnosis

After participants had returned their codings with respect to the first part of the case history, which gave the findings on initial assessment, they were sent the second part, which gave clinical information obtained during the period of follow-up. A further form was completed in which the participants had the opportunity to amend their original diagnosis on the first axis.

In only 3 cases (1, 9, and 10) did as many as one-third of the participants change their diagnosis, and in 6 cases none of the participants did so.

In case 1 (the boy showing severe aggression at home only) participants mainly changed their diagnosis from neurotic disorder to conduct disorder. Follow-up information showed that the boy's aggressive and destructive behaviour had persisted. Although this had always been a feature of the case many of the participants had at first made a diagnosis of neurotic disorder. Etiological considerations probably played some part in this judgement, although the codes were supposed to have been based solely on phenomenology. However, the persistence of aggression at follow-up seems to have led participants to use a more phenomenologically based code.

In case 9 the follow-up findings included the development of paranoid delusions, and many participants changed their diagnosis from personality disorder to psychosis.

In case 10 (a retarded child with a variety of behavioural difficulties), the persistence of tantrums into adolescence was associated with a shift from a neurotic disorder coding to one of either conduct disorder or personality disorder.

It may be concluded, from the infrequency with which first axis codings were changed, that in most cases a diagnosis of the clinical psychiatric syndrome may be made at the time of initial assessment. This is an important finding, as it would be a major drawback if cases could not be classified until after a period of follow-up. However, the diagnosis of conduct disorder was an exception. In both cases 1 and 10 the diagnostic coding was changed at follow-up in spite of the fact that the children's behaviour persisted without appreciable alteration. There seemed to be some reluctance to code conduct disorder unless socially disapproved behaviour persisted over a prolonged period. This requirement had no place in the glossary instructions, so it may be presumed that either value judgements or etiological considerations were influencing what was supposed to be a phenomenological coding. There are implications here concerning the need both for training in the use of a new classification scheme and also for precise, full, and unambiguous glossary instructions.

Difficulties in coding

First axis—clinical psychiatric syndrome

With any classification, difficulties in coding may arise from anomalies in the definition of syndromes, inadvertent ambiguities in instructions for coding, and unintended gaps—i.e., lack of a proper place to classify certain conditions (13). In an attempt to pin-point these difficulties participants were asked to note (on a special part of the coding form) whenever there were difficulties on either the ICD or MAS in coding a diagnosis (describing the nature of the difficulties when they occurred). Purely clinical difficulties in making a diagnostic formulation were excluded.

The participants were united in preferring the MAS as a whole, both because of its more specific orientation to the disorders of childhood and because of its superior handling of cases where psychiatric disorders were associated with either intellectual retardation or a medical condition. They also preferred the opportunity to differentiate between phenomenology and etiology that was provided by the MAS but not the ICD. The complaints concerning the ICD largely centred around the lack of differentiation provided by the global "behaviour disorder" category of 308 and the lack of other suitable categories for children's disorders. Because the complaints about the ICD with respect to children's disorders were so general and so pervasive and because they did not necessarily give rise to "difficulties" (it is easy, but not very fruitful, to code all cases 308), many of the complaints were not repeated for each individual case. For this reason, it is not particularly useful to compare the number of difficulties reported per case for each diagnostic scheme. There were 9 cases in which more difficulties were reported with the ICD and 5 in which there were more with the MAS (in the others there was an equal number of difficulties). This was reflected in a somewhat higher total of difficulties with the ICD in the series as a whole, but the difference fell just short of the 5% level of significance.

It is more useful to consider the nature of the difficulties encountered with each system, as there were clear differences between them. For this purpose the case material can usefully be divided into: (a) clear-cut disorders of a type well recognized in adult life; (b) disorders that are unique to childhood; (c) conditions in which psychiatric abnormality is closely associated with a physical or cognitive disorder; and (d) miscellaneous cases.

(a) Adult-type disorders

Where there was a clear-cut functional psychosis, as in case 14 (schizophrenic state in an adolescent) no difficulties were experienced with either system. Where there were well-defined neurotic disorders (depression—case 5, conversion hysteria—case 2, dog phobia—case 3) few difficulties were experienced with the ICD. Inter-rater agreement was also good on the MAS, but many participants wanted subdivisions within the neurotic category (only a single coding was provided). Similarly, there were very few difficulties with the ICD in the one case of sexual deviation, which fitted well into adult-type disorders. However, the MAS did not provide a separate coding for sexual deviation and most participants felt that one was necessary. In summary, the ICD was well suited (and better suited than the MAS) to clear-cut single disorders of an adult type.

The child with school refusal (case 8) was somewhat similar in that nearly all participants diagnosed neurotic disorder on both classification systems. Some participants expressed the opinion that this was a sufficiently distinctive syndrome to warrant a separate code under neurotic disorder in the MAS.

(b) Disorders of childhood

The situation was reversed in the case of disorders more typical of childhood. The MAS was well suited to cases of infantile autism (case 13), hyperkinetic disorder (case 6), and delinquency (case 17), whereas there was no appropriate coding in the ICD for any of these conditions. The MAS was also more suitable for the case of tearfulness in a young child (case 7) and the case of a child presenting with regressive behaviour and tantrums in association with a family crisis over the disposal of a mentally retarded sibling (case 15). In all of these cases, the experimental system worked better, not because of its multi-axial nature but because better provision had been made for child psychiatric disorders.

(c) Disorders associated with physical disease

The specific advantages of the MAS were most evident with the more complicated disorders such as case 11 (the girl with subacute sclerosing leucoencephalitis presenting as dementia with psychotic features), where the ICD forced a choice between making a coding describing the clinical features (293) or one describing the neurological disorder (323).[a] Of course, both could have been coded, but because the ICD does not specify this possibility most participants only coded one. The MAS allowed both categories to be coded on

---

[a] In fact, the correct coding on the ICD according to the alphabetical index is 065 (arthropod-borne viral disease), which merely emphasizes the confusion; no participant made this coding.

different axes. The same applied to case 13, in which infantile autism had developed on the basis of a luetic infection. Some participants made an ICD coding on the basis of etiology (i.e., congenital syphilis), some on the basis of intellectual level, some on the basis of the type of psychosis, some on the basis of a psychosis associated with organic brain syndrome, and some on the basis of various combinations of these. The MAS ensured that the psychiatric syndrome, intellectual level, and medical condition were all coded in the same systematic order by all participants.

(d) Miscellaneous difficulties

Neither system posed much difficulty in the case of encopresis (case 13). However, there were more complaints concerning the ICD, apparently because the category 306 referred to specific symptoms rather than specific disorders. A simple change of heading would remove this difficulty. The complaints about the MAS concerned the inclusion of encopresis within the developmental disorder category. Some participants thought that it would be better placed under a separate heading.

There were also a number of cases that posed some difficulties with respect to both systems of classification. The case of the mentally retarded girl with mild behavioural disturbance (case 10) was difficult to code, largely because of clinical uncertainty about how much behavioural disturbance could be regarded as intrinsic to the mental retardation and hence how much disturbance was required to merit a separate coding. Cases 1 and 9 were both clinically complex cases with a mixture of symptoms that did not readily fit into any one category. Participants expressed the view that a category of mixed emotional and conduct disorder would have helped. This was not available in either classification scheme. The child with epilepsy and a long history of conduct disorder presenting with an acute confusional state due to petit mal status (case 12) posed an exceptionally complicated problem. In this case the coding difficulties largely stemmed from uncertainty as to whether to give more weight to the acute or to the chronic disorder.

For case 11 (the child with a dementing process), some participants noted that there was a possible confusion between a coding of dementia and one of disintegrative psychosis. While there is some possibility of overlap, disintegrative psychosis is not always associated with dementia, the diagnosis being based on behavioural rather than intellectual changes. Furthermore, dementia need not be accompanied by any psychotic disturbance.

Second axis—intellectual level

There were very few difficulties in using the second axis of the MAS. In the only 5 cases where difficulties were reported, these concerned either what to do when cognitive tests showed wide variations in score (e.g., where performance tests gave an average score but verbal tests a retarded score) or how to code cases in which there was a changing IQ due to intellectual deterioration. In addition, some participants noted that it was desirable to be able to code very superior intelligence separately from average intelligence.

Third axis—biological factors

Most cases provided no difficulty in coding biological factors but problems arose in a few. Case 6 (the boy with the hyperkinetic syndrome) caused the most difficulties. He was mildly retarded but showed delayed motor milestones in infancy and still had some defect in fine motor coordination. There was also a history of threatened miscarriage during the pregnancy. However, there were no unequivocal abnormalities on neurological examination. As a result participants were divided as to how to code this case and expressed a need for a coding of "minimal cerebral dysfunction" or "non-specific neurological abnormality".

Case 12 posed difficulties only in so far as participants wished to specify the type of epilepsy (which was not provided for). For case 13 some participants would have liked to code more than one biological factor. Case 14 caused coding confusion for some participants due to the fact that developmental disorders could appear on either the first or the third axis. This seems to be an undesirable feature of the MAS.

Fourth axis—psychosocial factors

There were considerable problems with the fourth axis and in half the cases a majority of participants expressed difficulties in coding psychosocial factors. In nearly all instances the main problem was the expressed need to code more than one psychosocial factor.

Some of the participants found that the categories reflected a conceptual system that was foreign to them, and that there were no equivalents for what they felt were the meaningful psychosocial determinants. Another comment frequently voiced was that the fourth axis did not allow for the coding of parental personality or psychiatric disorder as an influential factor. It was also thought that some aspects of the fourth axis might apply to one parent while a quite different or contrary factor operated with respect to the other parent, e.g., an overprotective mother and a rejecting or hostile father.

Multiple coding

It has already been noted that most participants felt the need to code more than one psychosocial factor in at least some cases. Participants were also asked to note systematically those instances where they considered that more than one code was necessary on the first axis.

In most cases one or two participants wanted to use more than one coding for the clinical psychiatric syndrome but in only 5 cases did as many as a quarter wish to do so. In two cases (4 and 9) this was because clinicians wished to code both the presenting disorder and an associated personality disorder. These cases (both adolescents) gave rise to discussion as to whether it was more appropriate to consider personality disorder as a separate dimension of diagnosis rather than as an alternative to some acute psychiatric state. It was considered by most that a separate axis for personality was called for but that this issue arose in the case of only a few children and was more generally applicable to adults. Case 12 posed similar problems, illustrating the need to code both the presenting acute confusional state and the long-standing conduct disorder.

Cases 1 and 6 presented different problems; some participants wished to code different aspects of the *same* disorder (namely neurotic and conduct elements in Case 6). In other words, the problem was how to code mixed disorders rather than how to code associated disorders.

General remarks

The case-history exercise or some similar technique is invaluable for assessing inter-rater reliability. However, the restricted number of cases and the structured presentation of case material impose limitations on its usefulness in looking at other attributes of a classification system.

The small number of cases in a reliability exercise may lead to neglect of infrequently used, but nevertheless important, codings. The discriminating powers of a classification scheme also become most apparent when the system is applied to a large number of cases. If a particular code is used for an unduly high proportion of patients it is likely that the discrimination offered by that coding is inadequate.

Case histories will usually have been chosen on the basis of adequate information for classification. In order to determine whether such information is routinely available it is necessary to test the scheme in ordinary clinical practice. Furthermore, the content of the case material will inevitably influence the choice of factors that make up a diagnostic formulation. In studying the advantages of the MAS we are interested in the extent to which information relating to intellectual, organic, and psychosocial factors can be retrieved from a classification coding. By emphasizing or excluding information on these factors in a case history we inevitably influence the extent to which they will be noted.

The extent to which diagnostic categories are associated with differences in symptomatology, age and sex distribution, family background, treatment, and prognosis is also better assessed from a clinical study than from a case history exercise.

Accordingly, the ICD and MAS were compared with respect to a large series of ordinary clinic cases. All participants were asked to diagnose 10–15 successive new referrals to their own clinics on both the ICD and the MAS. They were asked to rate symptom severity, to detail their proposed treatment, and to give a social and symptomatic prognosis. Comments on coding difficulties were invited. Participants were also asked to follow up cases 6 months and 12 months after the child had first attended and, where necessary in the light of information available to them at that time, to revise their original diagnostic coding. Schedules were completed on 255 new cases and follow-up reports at 6 months or 12 months or both were obtained on 212 of these.

Characteristics of cases

Some of the characteristics of the 255 cases are given in Table 13 according to the diagnosis made on the first axis of the MAS.

Four diagnoses accounted for three-quarters of the cases. "Neurotic disorder" and "conduct disorder" were most frequently diagnosed (79 and 61 cases respectively). "Developmental disorder" was the next most frequent diagnosis (35 cases) and there were 25 cases of "adaptation reaction". All the other main codings were used in at least 8 cases, apart from "normal variation", which was used 5 times, and "psychosomatic" disorder, which was used only once. The last finding is particularly striking as 51 cases had been referred by paediatricians and 72 cases by family doctors.

As reported in most studies of clinic referrals, there was a majority of boys (60%), most children were in the middle age group of 5–11 years (58%), and a high proportion (30%) came from "broken homes" (i.e., were not living with their two natural parents).

Also in keeping with the findings of previous investigations, conduct disorders were particularly common in boys and were most frequently associated with "broken homes". Psychoses, mental retardation, developmental disorders, and, to a lesser extent, adaptation reactions were most characteristic of the younger age group.

TABLE 13
CHARACTERISTICS OF CLINICAL CASES

MAS 1st axis coding	Age (years)			Sex		Family situation		Total
	5	5–11	12+	M	F	Normal	"Broken"	
Normal variation	0	3	2	5	0	2	3	5
Adaptation reaction	5	16	4	15	10	15	10	25
Development disorder	9	23	3	26	9	25	10	35
Conduct disorder	1	31	29	45	16	30	29	61
Neurotic disorder	5	50	24	36	43	63	15	79
Psychosis	3	5	0	5	3	7	1	8
Personality disorder	0	8	5	7	6	8	5	13
"Psychosomatic" disorder	0	1	0	0	1	1	0	1
Other	0	4	5	4	5	9	0	9
Manifestation of mental retardation only	12	7	0	9	10	15	4	19
Total	35	148	72	153	102	176	77	255

Parallels between the ICD and the first axis codings of the MAS

Ten different first axis codes (including subdivisions of the first digit) were used to designate 5 or more cases out of the total group of 255 patients. Ten codes were used to describe 4 or fewer patients and 4 codes were not used at all. In Table 14 the 10 most frequently used first axis codes have been listed alongside those two ICD codes with which the given first axis code had been most frequently applied.

One code (308, behaviour disorders of childhood) was the most frequent ICD equivalent of no fewer than 6 of the 10 first axis MAS codes. MAS codings for which 308 was used as first equivalent were adaptation reaction, hyperkinetic disorder, conduct disorder, neurotic disorder, infantile psychosis, and personality disorder—a most diverse group of disorders of differing etiology, phenomenology, and prognosis. Although 37 of the 69 cases of neurotic disorder received one of the ICD diagnoses of neurosis in the 300 3-digit grouping, 40 had been coded 308. One first axis code (normal variation) had no ICD equivalent, and only two MAS codes had a meaningful ICD equivalent—specific learning disorder (306.1) and mental retardation (311). Thus, in spite of the much greater variety of ICD codes that were available for use, in practice they proved to be less discriminating for child psychiatric disorders than the MAS codes.

TABLE 14
ICD EQUIVALENTS OF MAS FIRST AXIS DIAGNOSIS

MAS 1st axis code			Most frequently used ICD code			2nd most frequently used ICD code		
Code		Total N	Code	No.	(%)	Code	No.	(%)
Neurotic disorder	(4.0)	79	308	40	51	300.0	14	18
Conduct disorder	(3.0)	61	308	49	80	301.7	10	16
Adaptation reaction	(1.0)	25	308	12	48	307	11	44
Manifestation of subnormality only	(9.0)	19	311.0	4	21	311.5	3	16
Personality disorder	(6.0)	13	308	6	46	306.1	3	23
Hyperkinetic disorder	(2.1)	9	308	4	44	311.0	4	44
Specific learning disorder	(2.3)	9	306.1	7	78	311.0	2	22
Other unspecified disorders	(8.5)	6	300.0	2	33	307	2	33
Normal variation	(0.0)	6	No ICD equivalent					
Infantile psychosis	(5.1)	5	308	2	40	299.9	2	40

The poor discrimination of the ICD code 308 is also shown by the reverse procedure, illustrated in Table 15, namely listing the first axis equivalents of the 6 most commonly used ICD codes. Code 308 was used with 120 cases—58% of the total sample. This is a much higher proportion of the sample than that covered by the most frequently used MAS first axis code (neurotic disorder, used in 31% of cases). The 308 code was used with no fewer than 14 different first axis codes, which again shows the lack of differentiation provided by this coding.

TABLE 15
MAS FIRST AXIS EQUIVALENTS OF ICD DIAGNOSES

ICD code			Most frequently used with first axis			2nd most frequently used with first axis	
Code		Total N	Code	No.	(%)	Code	(%)
Behaviour disorder of childhood	(308)	120	3	49	41	4	33
Anxiety neurosis	(300.0)	23	4	14	61	1	4
Depressive neurosis	(300.4)	19	4	10	53	3	21
Transient situational disorder	(307)	17	1	11	23	4	12
Specific learning disorder	(306.1)	16	2.3	7	44	4	19
Antisocial personality disorder	(307.1)	13	3	10	77	6	15

As was shown in the case-history exercise, this table also demonstrates that the ICD codings for neurosis provide better differentiation than does the equivalent single-category MAS code. "Anxiety neurosis" and "depressive neurosis" can be differentiated on the former but not on the latter scheme. "Transient situational disorder" (367) has a fair equivalent in "adaptation reaction", and the code for "specific learning disorder" is present in both systems. In cases where an ICD diagnosis of "antisocial personality disorder" (301.7) was made, the first axis code of conduct disorder was nearly always given as classifying individual clinical cases. At the completion of the study two meetings

Difficulties in using the two schemes

Participants were asked to list the difficulties they had experienced in classifying individual clinical cases. At the completion of the study two meetings were held, attended by the majority of the participants. Note was taken of further difficulties mentioned during the discussion.

An assessment of the difficulties noted at the time of coding showed that significantly more difficulties were reported in using the ICD than in using the MAS. Difficulties in coding were reported for 65 cases on the MAS and for 114 cases on the ICD.

The frequency with which such difficulties were associated with different diagnostic categories is presented in Table 16.

TABLE 16
DIFFICULTIES IN USING THE TWO SCHEMES

Disorder[a]		No.	Difficulties	
			MAS (%)	ICD (%)
Neurotic disorder	(4.0)	79	36	49
Conduct disorder	(3.0)	61	28	49
Adjustment reaction	(1.0)	25	24	60
Personality disorder	(6.0)	13	38	31
Hyperkinetic disorder	(2.1)	9	22	78
Specific learning disorder	(2.3)	9	44	11
Other unspecified disorders	(8.5)	6	100	67
Infantile psychosis	(5.1)	5	—	100
No psychiatric disorder	(0.0)	5	0	80
Total			65 (cases)	114 (cases)

[a] Code 9 and codes used infrequently have been omitted from this table.

The greater problems with the ICD were most evident in connexion with the diagnoses most characteristic of childhood—adaptation reaction, hyperkinetic disorder, conduct disorder, and infantile psychosis. However, where there was an ICD code for such childhood disorders, as in the case of specific learning difficulties, no greater difficulties were experienced with the ICD. With the two major diagnostic categories of neurotic disorder and personality disorder, difficulties occurred with about the same frequency in the two systems. The nature of the difficulties is discussed below.

Normal variation

Normal variation gave rise to no difficulties in the MAS but there were problems with the ICD in that no code was provided for this diagnosis.

Adaptation reaction

This category was used to describe both mild conditions of good prognosis and also conditions thought to be reactions to acutely stressful life situations. The nearest ICD equivalent—transient situational disturbance—was used somewhat less frequently and was defined solely in terms of reaction to stress. The glossary suggested that it should be restricted to very short-lived acute reactions to stress, which makes it inapplicable to most of the cases for which the MAS code of "adaptation reaction" was used.

Developmental disorders

On the whole this category gave rise to relatively few serious difficulties in coding on the first axis. Specific learning difficulties posed few problems but, as with other developmental disorders, there were difficulties in coding when such a condition was also associated with an emotional disorder. The glossary provided instructions on what to do in this situation, but evidently they were inadequate or had not been understood. The code for hyperkinetic disorder was also reasonably adequate but it was noted that some cases included symptoms not specified in the glossary definition. Only one case of tics was recorded and here the clinician noted that it did not fit into the general definition of developmental disorder and suggested that the code for tics would be better placed elsewhere. In the discussion of this case at the meeting of participants it was also generally agreed that tics and Gilles de la Tourette's syndrome were not clearly distinguishable and so should not be coded under different headings.

Conduct disorders

The main coding difficulty noted in connexion with "conduct disorder" was the frequent occurrence of cases in which both neurotic and antisocial symptoms were present. Many participants noted that an appropriate coding should be available for this situation. Some also expressed unease about using a phenomenological diagnosis when it was thought that the symptoms had arisen on a "neurotic" basis. In discussion it was agreed that it was not possible in the present state of knowledge to include such theoretical considerations in an international classification. Nevertheless, it was seen that such considerations, in conjunction with the feeling that the term "conduct disorder" carried a pejorative connotation, had led some participants to put cases of stealing in the neurotic category. They thought that the more general term "disturbance of conduct" carried fewer prejudicial overtones than "conduct disorder", which illustrates the problem that changes in attitudes can be associated with even small changes in wording, and also reflects the difficulty in persuading clinicians to adhere to the operational definitions provided in a glossary rather than to follow their habitual usages of diagnostic terms.

Particularly in the case of adolescents, some difficulties were experienced in deciding when to code conduct disorder and when to code personality disorder. It was again noted that personality really constituted a different dimension from that covered by the clinical psychiatric syndrome. Some confusion between conduct disorder and hyperkinetic disorder occurred in a few cases.

All participants agreed that a further subdivision of conduct disorders was indicated.

Neurotic disorders

Here too, difficulties were experienced in coding cases with an admixture of emotional and conduct disturbance. Some had been coded as conduct disorder and some as neurotic disorder, without a clear indication of why one coding had been preferred to the other.

Several participants found difficulty in coding cases, particularly of young children, where temper tantrums or relationship difficulties were the most prominent feature.

It was pointed out that the presence in children of emotional disturbance could not be equated with adult neurosis and a preference was expressed for using emotional disorders (rather than neurotic disorders) as the main term.

Psychotic disorders

Few difficulties were experienced in connexion with psychotic disorders but it was noted that there was a need for a coding of depressive psychosis, particularly in the case of adolescents.

In discussion, it was also noted that there was a problem in coding cases where mental retardation was accompanied by psychotic features but where the disorder did not fulfil the criteria for infantile autism.

Personality disorders

Participants had difficulty in deciding whether to code conduct disorder or personality disorder in long-standing cases of disturbance. Also, they considered that a subdivision of personality disorders was required. It was noted that the diagnosis and coding of some of the more severe behavioural disturbances in epileptic children posed problems in that they did not readily fit into any of the codings provided.

Other disorders

The non-specific category "other disorders" was used for several cases of depression by one participant, who felt that no other coding was suitable. In discussion it was agreed that a specific coding for depressive disorders was required.

One case raised the problem of how to code disorders in older children where the original problem was one of hyperkinesis but where the overactivity had ceased as the child grew older. It was recognized that this was a common occurrence and that some means must be found of dealing with cases where the main problem is a disorder of attention and distractibility associated with overactivity in early childhood but normal or diminished activity in adolescence.

Mental retardation

Several participants were unsure how to decide what degree of behavioural disturbance could be expected as part of mental retardation and what degree warranted a separate coding for one or other clinical psychiatric syndrome.

Difficulties in using the second axis

Difficulties experienced with the second axis (intellectual level) were similar to those noted during the first part of the study. In particular, there was uncertainty how to code when different IQ tests produced widely varying scores.

Difficulties in using the third axis

When the third axis was being designed it had been decided to emphasize the medical conditions that were present at the time the child attended the clinic rather than disorders that had occurred only in the past. Thus, in the case of cerebral palsy due to perinatal damage the cerebral palsy would be coded and not the perinatal damage. The practical advantages (and greater reliability) of this approach were accepted by most participants, but a few thought that it should be possible to code biological factors that *might* have had an influence on development, even when these factors were no longer active.

For the same reasons, some participants regretted that it was not possible to code in accordance with their view that a disorder was genetically determined. However, it was recognized that such a procedure was incompatible with the coding of medical conditions and, in any case, introduced judgements on which psychiatrists were unlikely to agree.

Some felt that it should be possible to code pregnancy and puberty as states (but not disorders) that might be relevant to the psychiatric disorder.

It was generally considered necessary to be able, under the general heading of epilepsy, to code the type of fit.

Difficulties were also experienced from the inclusion of developmental disorders on both the first and third axes.

Multiple coding

One of the theoretical advantages of the MAS is that it ensures uniformity of practice both in which aspects of a case receive a coding and in which order codings are made, thus permitting easy comparability of codings between different centres. However, the ICD allows multiple codings and if clinicians used these in a similar fashion there would be no need for the structure of a MAS. By comparing ICD and MAS codes, it was possible to determine how far this occurred in the present study with respect to medical conditions and mental retardation.

There were 68 cases in which a coding of a medical condition (other than a developmental disorder) was made on the third axis. In 21 cases (31%) this was not noted in terms of any ICD code. In an additional 13 cases the medical condition was indicated only imprecisely in terms of the fourth digit of the mental retardation code. Thus, in nearly a third of cases the ICD made no note of the medical condition and in a further sixth it was noted only very imprecisely. Of the 21 cases of medical conditions that were missed, 12 concerned diseases of the central nervous system or special senses (such as cerebral palsy, epilepsy, blindness, or deafness) that were likely to be of considerable psychiatric importance.

When a medical condition was noted in the ICD coding its coding position was unpredictable. When the condition was noted in a separate ICD code, it appeared as the first code twice, the second code 7 times, and third code twice. When the condition was recorded in the mental retardation combination code it appeared in the first position 23 times and the second position twice.

The same was true of mental retardation; of the 27 cases of mild mental retardation noted on the second axis, only 15 were noted in terms of any ICD code, i.e., 44% were missed by the ICD coding. Of the 15 cases that did receive an ICD coding, the mental retardation code appeared in the first position 11 times and in the second position 4 times.

Fewer cases of moderate or severe mental retardation were missed but the position of the coding was equally unpredictable. Of the 22 cases of moderate, severe, or profound mental retardation, 2 (10%) were missed. Of the 20 cases recorded, the mental retardation coding appeared first 16 times, second once, and third 3 times. The one case in which the level of mental retardation could not be estimated was not noted in the ICD coding. These findings are summarized in Tables 17 and 18.

TABLE 17
ICD CODING WHEN A MEDICAL CONDITION WAS NOTED ON THE THIRD AXIS

	Total No.	Missed by ICD	1st position	2nd position	3rd position
Disorder of CNS or special senses	49	13	25	9	2
Other medical conditions	19	8	3	5	3
Total	68	21	28	14	5

TABLE 18
ICD CODING WHEN MENTAL RETARDATION WAS NOTED ON THE SECOND AXIS

	Total No.	Missed by ICD	1st position	2nd position	3rd position
Mild retardation	27	12	11	4	0
Moderate retardation	14	2	8	1	3
Severe/profound retardation	8	0	8	0	0
Level not estimated	1	1	0	0	0
Total	50	15	27	5	3

In short, it was evident that because the ICD specified neither which aspects of a case should be coded nor the order in which the codings should be made, it failed to record serious and clinically important medical conditions, and it failed to record mental retardation. If the analysis of ICD codes were restricted to the first coding, the error rate would be even higher, because when codes were made they might appear in the first, second, or third position.

Meaningfulness of the proposed categories

Some of the diagnostic categories used in the MAS are well established (such as infantile psychosis) or already have a coding in the ICD. Others require more empirical justification. This applies particularly to the new category of adaptation reaction. The concept of personality disorder as evident in childhood remains problematical and warrants examination. The subdivision of the general category of behavioural disorders into neurotic and conduct disorders is well supported by the results of previous studies (*16*) but the validity of the distinction can also be examined here. Some of the other categories (such as the hyperkinetic syndrome) also deserve study, but the number of such cases in the present investigation was too small for them to be considered.

The meaningfulness of the distinction between different diagnostic categories differed from one another in terms of criteria other than the diagnosis. The available criteria (age and sex distribution, symptomatology, family situation, duration of disorder, prognosis, treatment, and outcome) are considered below with respect to adaptation reaction, conduct disorder, neurotic disorder, and personality disorder.

Age and sex distribution

The children with an adaptation reaction differed from those with a conduct disorder by virtue of there being significantly more children under the age of 5 ($\chi^2 = 6.59$, $v^a = 1$, $P < .05$). Those with a conduct disorder were also somewhat older than the others but the difference fell short of statistical significance.

The main sex difference concerned the neurotic and conduct disorder groups. Three-quarters of the youngsters with a conduct disorder were boys, whereas in the neurotic group the sex ratio was approximately equal with a slight preponderance of girls. ($\chi^2 = 10.10$; $v = 1$; $P < .01$). This finding is in keeping with those of previous studies (*18*).

TABLE 19
AGE AND SEX DISTRIBUTION IN FOUR DIAGNOSTIC GROUPS

	Diagnosis			
	Adaptation reaction (%)	Conduct disorder (%)	Neurotic disorder (%)	Personality disorder (%)
Age (years)	(N = 25)	(N = 61)	(N = 79)	(N = 13)
< 5	20	2	6	0
5–11	64	51	63	61
12 or over	16	47	30	38
Sex distribution				
Boys (%)	60	74	46	54

Family situation

Most of the children in the neurotic group were living with their two natural parents and only 19% were in homes "broken" by death, divorce, or separation of the parents. The rate of "broken homes" was high in all three other groups, being highest in the conduct disorder group (47%), which differed significantly from the neurotic group in this respect ($\chi^2 = 11.73$; $v = 1$; $P < .001$). The adaptation reaction and personality disorder groups had rates of "broken

---

[a] v = the number of degrees of freedom.

homes" (40% and 38% respectively) nearly as high as those of the conduct disorder group.

Symptomatology

Certain symptoms, such as disturbed family relationships, were recorded for the vast majority of cases and were of no value in differential diagnosis. Others, such as hyperkinesis or stereotypies, did differentiate diagnoses but only with respect to rarer conditions. Five symptoms significantly differentiated the four commoner disorders under consideration.

Children with a conduct disorder were less likely than those in any of the other three diagnostic groups to be rated as showing emotional disturbance. They were also somewhat less likely to have disturbed relationships with their peers. As was to be expected, they more often showed antisocial behaviour, but in this respect they closely resembled the children with personality disorder. Somatic symptoms were very common in those with personality disorder and they occurred in a third of the neurotic children, but they were distinctly uncommon in both the other groups. Educational retardation was common to all four diagnostic groups but was present particularly in the children with personality disorder, who received this rating in 85% of cases. The severity of disturbance could be roughly assessed by comparing the mean symptom rating for the four groups. The mean symptom rating was 4.0 for children with an adaptation reaction, 4.2 for those with a conduct disorder,[a] 4.7 for those with a neurotic disorder, and 6.2 for those with a personality disorder.

TABLE 20
SYMPTOMATOLOGY IN FOUR DIAGNOSTIC GROUPS

| | Diagnosis | | | |
Symptoms	Adaptation reaction (% with symptom)	Conduct disorder (% with symptom)	Neurotic disorder (% with symptom)	Personality disorder (% with symptom)
Emotional disturbance	83	67	95	100
Disturbed peer relationships	80	69	85	86
Antisocial behaviour	40	76	38	70
Somatic symptoms	12	11	35	61
Educational retardation	40	49	42	85

Duration of disorder

The duration of the disorder was assessed on a 5-point scale, 0 denoting a duration of less than 6 months, 1 a duration of 6–11 months, 2 a duration of 12–23 months, 3 a duration of 24–35 months, and 4 a duration of 36 months or more. Differences in duration between the four diagnostic groups were compared by means of the mean rating on this scale. Duration was shortest for the children with an adaptation reaction (mean score 2.00) or a conduct disorder (mean score 2.17) and longest for those with a personality disorder (mean score 3.17), the difference between personality disorder and adaptation reaction being significant at the 1% level ($t = 2.761$; $v = 33$) and the difference between per-

---

[a] The mean score for children with conduct disorder was artefactually low because only one symptom coding was provided for socially disapproved behaviour.

sonality disorder and conduct disorder being significant at the 5% level ($t = 2.585$, $v = 68$). Neurotic disorders occupied an intermediate position ($t = 2.61$).

Prognosis

Prognosis was rated separately for symptoms and for social adjustment, each being on a 4-point scale ranging from 0 for no symptoms and normal social adjustment to 3 for severe symptoms and severe difficulties in adjustment. The participants were asked to predict the child's state one year after the initial clinical assessment.

TABLE 21
PROGNOSIS IN FOUR DIAGNOSTIC GROUPS

	Diagnosis			
Prognosis	Adaptation reaction (mean score)	Conduct disorder (mean score)	Neurotic disorder (mean score)	Personality disorder (mean score)
Symptoms	0.88	1.63	1.36	2.20
Social adjustment	0.94	1.63	1.46	2.22

The prognosis given to children with a personality disorder was poor with respect to both symptoms ($t = 2.785$; $v = 37$; $P < .01$) and social adjustment ($t = 4.538$; $v = 34$; $P < .001$), and significantly worse in both cases than the prognosis given to children with an adaptation reaction. The children with a conduct disorder and those with a neurotic disorder occupied an intermediate position in both cases and these two groups did not differ from each other.

Treatment

Case work or psychotherapy with the parents was proposed for about half of all cases, irrespective of diagnosis. Supportive treatment was recommended equally often and this, too, did not differentiate the groups. Psychotherapy with the child was advised most frequently in the case of youngsters with a personality disorder (77% of cases) and least often for those with an adaptation reaction (40% of cases) but none of the inter-group differences was significant. Behaviour therapy was scarcely ever used (less than 5% of cases), inpatient care infrequently (0–15% of cases, according to diagnosis), and drugs were prescribed in about a third of cases, irrespective of diagnosis (with a range from 20% in children with conduct disorder to 30% in those with a personality disorder). The only treatments that differed significantly with diagnosis were special schooling and residential placement.

TABLE 22
SPECIAL SCHOOLING AND RESIDENTIAL TREATMENT IN FOUR DIAGNOSTIC GROUPS

	Diagnosis			
Recommended treatment	Adaptation reaction (%)	Conduct disorder (%)	Neurotic disorder (%)	Personality disorder (%)
Special schooling	25	26	20	77
Residential placement	8	26	9	46

Residential placement was recommended more frequently for children with conduct disorders than for neurotic children. ($\chi^2 = 6.35$; $v = 1$; $P < .05$). Youngsters with personality disorders were significantly more likely to be recommended for special schooling than children in other diagnostic categories, the greatest contrast being with neurotic disorder ($\chi^2 = 14.99$; $v = 1$; $P < .001$). Nearly half (46%) of the children with personality disorders were recommended for residential placement.

Outcome

The outcome as measured at one year followed the initial prediction quite closely. The children with an adaptation reaction had done very well with respect to both symptomatology and social adjustment, and the personality

TABLE 23
OUTCOME IN FOUR DIAGNOSTIC GROUPS

Outcome	Diagnosis			
	Adaptation reaction	Conduct disorder	Neurotic disorder	Personality disorder
Mean symptom score	0.50	1.10	1.52	1.77
Mean social adjustment score	0.63	1.92	1.22	2.10

disorder children had done badly in both areas, the differences in outcome between these categories being statistically significant (symptom state $t = 2.398$; $v = 23$; $P < .05$; social adjustment $t = 3.852$; $v = 28$; $P < .001$). The conduct disorder and neurotic disorder groups occupied an intermediate position in both respects but although the differences fell short of significance it is noticeable that the pattern differed between the groups. The neurotic children still had a moderate level of symptoms but their degree of social adjustment was rather better. By contrast, the children with conduct disorders had few symptoms but their social adjustment was poor, being nearly as bad as that for the personality disorder group.

Change of diagnosis

Clinicians were asked to note any changes of diagnosis when the cases were reviewed at the 6-months and 12-months follow-ups. Of the original group of 252 cases, follow-up information was available at one or other follow-up examination in 212 cases (at one year follow-up in 171 of these). In only 16 cases were there changes in diagnostic coding. The changes followed no particular pattern except that they were somewhat more frequent in neurotic children, who accounted for 7 of the 16 cases, and that a third of the changes were to adaptation reaction (5). This is in line with the conclusion above that such a diagnosis is made mainly on the basis of actual or expected outcome.

Mental retardation

One of the chief characteristics of the MAS is that it records the clinical psychiatric syndrome and the intellectual level separately. The rationale for this procedure is that both are important aspects of diagnosis, that psychiatric disorder and mental retardation are frequently associated, and that, with the exception of certain rarer disorders, the form of psychiatric disorder is not predictable from the knowledge that the patient is retarded (19). It was possible to examine each of these issues with regard to the cases in the present series.

Of the total of 252 patients, 51 were coded on the second axis as showing some degree of mental retardation. In 19 cases the retardation was not associated with a psychiatric disorder but in the remaining 32 cases some clinical psychiatric syndrome was recorded. As in the children of normal intelligence, neurotic disorder was the commonest diagnosis, with a rate of 33%. Conduct disorder was less frequent than in the series as a whole but it was coded twice (6% of cases). Personality disorder was noted three times, a rate (9%) very slightly above that for children of normal intelligence. An adaptation reaction was noted once (3% of cases). Thus, the common emotional and behavioural disturbances that accounted for 80% of disorders in children of normal intelligence also accounted for just half of the psychiatric disorders seen in mentally retarded children.

TABLE 24
PSYCHIATRIC DISORDER IN CHILDREN OF NORMAL AND SUBNORMAL INTELLIGENCE

Diagnosis	Mentally retarded children		Other children	
	(No.)	(%)	(No.)	(%)
Adaptation reaction	1	3	24	12
Hyperkinetic disorder	7	22	2	1
Conduct disorder	2	6	59	29
Neurotic disorder	11	34	68	34
Infantile psychosis	5	15	0	0
Personality disorder	3	9	10	5
Other	3	9	38	19
Total	32		201	

The main difference lay in the diagnoses of hyperkinetic disorder (made in 22% of retarded children as compared with 1% of children of normal intelligence) and infantile psychosis (made in 15% of retarded children and in none of those of normal intelligence). Although these accounted for only a minority of the psychiatric disorders among retarded children they were much more common (and significantly so) than in children who were not retarded.

Comparisons were also made between the mentally retarded with a psychiatric disorder and those without any coded disorder. There was a significant age difference between the groups. Only 19% of the retarded children with psychiatric disorder were under 5 years of age, whereas 63% of those without psychiatric disorder were under that age.

As expected, the groups differed in symptomatology, most symptoms being commoner in the psychiatric disorder group. Emotional disturbance, autism, disturbed family relationships, disturbed peer relationships, and antisocial behaviour were all significantly more common. However, there were no differences with respect to enuresis/encopresis, speech delay, sleeping/eating difficulties, and educational retardation, all of which occurred in the majority of retarded children, regardless of whether they were diagnosed as having a psychiatric disorder.

The children without psychiatric disorder were significantly more likely to be recommended for special schooling (74% and 22% respectively) but those with a disorder were significantly more likely to be given psychotherapy or drug treatment. Interestingly, there was no difference between the groups in symptomatology or social adjustment at the one-year follow-up; the intellectual level was therefore of greater prognostic value than was the presence of psychiatric disorder. The numbers were too small for statistical analysis but it seemed that the *type* of psychiatric disorder might be of greater prognostic importance in that the children with psychosis, hyperkinetic syndrome, and personality disorder showed particularly poor progress.

There is no simple association between intellectual retardation and psychiatric disorder. Both are crucial elements in the diagnosis and require separate coding. It is evident from the findings described earlier that if this is to be done systematically some form of multi-axial classification is necessary.

In summary, most of the previously reported differences between groups with neurotic and conduct disorders were replicated in the present study. The children with conduct disorder differed from those with neurotic disorder in being mostly boys who showed antisocial behaviour, few somatic complaints, and little emotional disturbance, who frequently came from "broken homes", who were quite often recommended for residential placement, and who, at follow-up a year later, tended to have a poor social adjustment but not many symptoms. These differences are sufficient to warrant separate categories for the two types of disturbances. However, the degree of overlap between the groups was considerable (for example, over a third of the neurotic children showed antisocial symptoms) and if the two categories are to be distinguished, obviously some provision must be made for a mixed type of disturbance.

The children with an adaptation reaction did not differ from other groups in terms of symptomatology, but they were distinguished by virtue of their mild symptoms, relatively short duration of disturbance, and good prognosis. It was also noticeable that a high proportion came from a disturbed family setting. The clinicians' good prognosis proved to be a valid prediction, in that one year later the children showed strikingly few symptoms and had a good social adjustment. It is clear from these findings that a group of children with mild transient disorder can be accurately defined. Accordingly, it would be possible to have a diagnostic coding based on the severity rather than on the type of symptomatology. The present findings suggest that such a category might be useful.

The personality disorder group tended to differ in the opposite direction in that there were many symptoms of long duration, and both the prognosis and actual outcome were poor. Symptoms of all types were very common but antisocial behaviour, somatic symptoms, and educational retardation were particularly so. It seems that this coding was mainly used for severe and persistent disorders with an admixture of emotional, educational, and antisocial disturbance.

The categories of hyperkinetic syndrome and infantile psychosis stood out as different from the others in terms of the frequent association with intellectual retardation. These categories also differed in terms of symptomatology and the children's poor outcome (both actual and predicted), but the numbers were too small for statistical analysis.

It may be concluded that the findings provide some support for the meaningfulness of most of the proposed main categories on the first axis of the MAS.

Information demands of the MAS

The clinical study clearly showed that sufficient information was regularly obtained in ordinary clinical practice, both inpatient and outpatient, for coding to be made on all four axes. The information demands for coding clinical psychiatric syndrome on the first axis were no different in kind from those already required by the ICD, and were easily met. The straightforward distinctions required for the second axis (intellectual level) were the same as those needed for ICD coding and did not necessarily require psychological testing. Obviously, testing is highly desirable if mental retardation is suspected but, in any case, this is routine practice in most clinics. The third axis is no more than a summary of ICD codings outside section V, so that coding on this axis, too, made no unusual information demands. The fourth axis proved unsatisfactory in the form used, but information on psychosocial influences is regularly obtained as part of any child psychiatric assessment, so that coding should present no difficulties once a satisfactory coding scheme is developed.

The suitability of the MAS for use in primary medical care (general practice) has not been assessed.

Statistical presentation of data from the MAS

The main purpose of a multi-axial scheme is to facilitate the collection of systematic information in a form that makes retrieval easy and comparative statistics reliable and valid. For most purposes it will be neither necessary nor desirable to present data from all four axes simultaneously. Obviously, the manner of presentation must vary with the purposes for which the data are required, but there are two types of questions that are likely to arise frequently and cannot be accurately answered on the basis of the Eighth Revision of the ICD: the number of cases of a particular type seen per specified time period, and the association between different disabilities.

The number of cases of a particular type seen per specified time period

Most commonly, statistics are required on the number of cases in a particular psychiatric category (e.g., neurotic disorder or infantile psychosis) seen during the course of one year (or some other time period). This information is readily obtained from the first axis codings, when, as in Table 13, the data are given by sex and by age distribution. Alternatively, information may be required regarding the number of cases with mental retardation, when the second axis may be used in the same way (as in the first column of Table 18). The same applies to the number of children with organic brain disorder, which is readily obtained by analysis of the third axis.

The principles of presentation in this respect are, of course, no different to those used with ICD-8. The really important difference, however, is that with the MAS it will be known that all cases have been coded (because there must be a coding on each axis), whereas this will not be so with ICD-8. With ICD-8 it is very probable (as the clinical study findings show) that if the child has a multiple problem only some aspects will be coded. Furthermore, it is quite uncertain in which order each element, if coded, will appear. Thus, with the MAS the intellectual level coding will always be found second, whereas in the ICD it may be first, second, third, fourth, fifth, or not present at all. In short, simple frequency counts are both easier and more valid with the MAS than with the ICD.

The association between different disabilities

Questions that may frequently arise are, for example: how many mentally retarded children also show some other psychiatric disorder?, or how does the distribution of psychiatric diagnoses vary between mentally retarded children and normally intelligent children? (as answered in Table 24), or what proportion of children with psychiatric disorder also have cerebral palsy or epilepsy? All that is required for these analyses is a straightforward cross-tabulation between two axes. Again, none of these questions could be reliably answered from ICD-8 because it would be unknown how often each of these elements had been coded when present. Furthermore, even if the missing information is ignored, cross-tabulations on ICD-8 are greatly complicated by the fact that each element to be compared may appear in any order among the codes used. This difficulty does not arise with the MAS.

In short, the statistical presentations of data from the MAS should be both very much easier and more reliable than is the case with ICD-8.

Implications for multi-axial classifications

The value of a multi-axial approach

The statistical analysis of findings from both the reliability study and the clinical study demonstrated the advantages of a multi-axial system of classification. The MAS scheme was much preferred by the study participants, both in theory and in practice. Participants found the multi-axial method easy to apply because it corresponded more closely to their approach in ordinary clinical practice. The separation of clinical psychiatric syndrome, intellectual level, associated physical disorders, and associated psychosocial factors on separate axes enabled a more unified system of coding to be carried out on each axis, provided fuller information about each case, and, furthermore, provided this information in a more systematic fashion that allowed better comparability between different centres.

The advantages were most clearly seen with respect to psychiatric disorders with an associated physical condition or with associated intellectual retardation. In both cases, ICD-8, as ordinarily used,[a] gave less information and gave even that information in a form that was not comparable between clinics or between cases. Thus, in only two-thirds of the 68 cases where some physical disorder was recorded on the third axis of the MAS was this noted in the ICD coding. Cases of spastic diplegia, blindness, deafness, asthma, and epilepsy were not reflected in the ICD coding even when these disorders were thought to be clinically significant in the psychiatrist's own diagnostic formulation. Of course, these physical conditions could have been coded on the ICD scheme but because there were no instructions on what clinical features to classify and how many codings to use, clinicians varied greatly in their practice. The same issue arose when psychiatric disorders were associated with intellectual retardation. On the ICD scheme the diagnosis of intellectual retardation was not always reflected in the codings. It too could have been coded, but because of the lack of instructions it was not coded systematically. A further difficulty stemmed from variation in the order used in ICD codings. Where there was both a psychiatric syndrome and intellectual retardation, clinicians varied in which they coded first. As many statistical analyses are still carried out using the first coding only, this would lead to both a loss of and non-comparability of information. Because the MAS provided a consistent and standard structure by which both intellectual retardation and physical disorder were always recorded in the same way, these problems could be avoided.

---

[a] As pointed out in the introduction, the ICD could be organized within a multi-axial framework if the appropriate coding instructions and other modifications were made. The comments here refer only to the use of ICD-8 as ordinarily employed without such a framework.

Further problems with respect to intellectual retardation arose because of the particular way in which the ICD-8 fourth digit in the mental retardation coding specifies hypothesized etiological influences rather than actual physical disorders or handicaps (as in the multi-axial scheme). In the first place the actual use of the fourth digit has been shown to be highly unreliable. In the second, it fails to make clinically important distinctions. Thus, the fourth digit coding of −.4 was used for both mental retardation of unknown etiology without accompanying physical handicap and for mental retardation associated with cerebral palsy. Similarly, the −.0 coding was used for cases of unknown origin, of rubella embryopathy, and of measles encephalitis.

A further important advantage of the MAS was the differentiation between the clinical psychiatric syndrome and the etiological influences. There was general agreement that this made classification both easier and more uniform in areas where psychiatrists are still not in agreement about theoretical issues concerning etiology.

For all these reasons it is clear that further work should be directed towards the possibility that in the future the ICD might be based on a multi-axial approach. This would constitute a change in structure and before such a change is made further research is needed on the merits and demerits of a multi-axial system as used in different cultures and with different groups of patients.

Modification of the ICD

Although it would be inappropriate to change the ICD to a multi-axial system at this stage, a few relatively minor alterations would remove many of the structural defects in section V of ICD-8 and would bring many of the advantages of a multi-axial approach without moving fully to a multi-axial system. Changes in the following areas would be sufficient to bring this about.

Mental retardation

The arrangement in ICD-8 for coding mental retardation provides only a crude fourth digit coding for the associated physical condition. The medical information given in this coding is quite inadequate in coverage and in addition has proved to be most unreliable (*11*). The defects in this arrangement could be removed if it ceased to be a combination category and if instructions were given to code any associated physical condition in a second coding from the appropriate sections of the ICD outside section V. This procedure would record the same information on the degree of intellectual impairment, and in addition there would be fuller and more systematic information on underlying or associated medical conditions.

Organic psychoses

The ICD-8 codings for organic psychoses (292–294 inclusive) provide no information on the type of psychiatric syndrome, and the differentiation of medical conditions is crude and inadequate. Thus, Huntington's chorea and multiple sclerosis receive the same coding (293.4), and so do hypoxia at birth, skull fracture, and surgical injury to the brain (293.5). This serious loss of information is a common feature of combination categories. These defects could also be largely overcome if combination categories were eliminated, if the section V coding specified the type of clinical psychiatric syndrome (e.g., dementia, acute confusional state, or depressive psychosis associated with organic brain pathology), and if instructions were given to code the associated physical condition more accurately than at present by means of the appropriate ICD coding outside section V. Similar proposals have been made by Wing (*13*), Essen-Möller (*12*), and Helmchen (*36*) in discussions of multi-axial schemes on the basis of other research.

Presumably disorders of physical psychogenic origin

The ICD-8 category 305 for physical disorder of presumably psychogenic origin has proved most unsatisfactory in that it overlaps with hysterical neurosis on the one hand and with a wide range of disorders in other sections of the ICD on the other. Thus, peptic ulcer may be coded under 305.5 or 532 and asthma under 305.2 or 493. Furthermore, the physical disorders in 305 are grouped by means of body system. The result is that it is not possible to differentiate between aerophagy, cyclical vomiting, peptic ulcer, and ulcerative colitis—conditions with an entirely different pathological basis. As in the other two areas where this problem arises, the difficulty could be overcome by coding the psychiatric aspect of the problem under 305 (or somewhere else in section V) and by giving instructions that the physical condition be more accurately and more appropriately covered by a code from the relevant section of the ICD outside section V.

The particular axes included in the MAS

Intellectual level

The second axis (intellectual level) was generally needed and on the whole it gave rise to a few difficulties. Some questions were raised about the need for more detailed instructions in the glossary to deal with various specific points. These points are dealt with below in the discussion on the modification of the ICD for child psychiatric disorders.

Biological factors

The third axis (biological factors) consisted simply of a summary of the whole of ICD-8, with a few additions and modifications. Accordingly, any criticisms apply more to ICD-8 than to the MAS as such. Nevertheless it is convenient to consider the points here. On the whole, few difficulties were found in either the reliability study or the clinical study. The two main problems concerned epilepsy and non-specific neurological syndromes. The third axis did not provide for a subdivision of epilepsy according to the type of fit; and this was generally felt to be necessary. ICD-8 does provide a subdivision into different varieties of epilepsy but the particular subdivisions provided are not entirely satisfactory. It is suggested that psychomotor fits should be separated from Jacksonian attacks, that myoclonic epilepsy and major fits should be differentiated, and that the category for petit mal should not include other varieties of minor fit. The other problem arose with non-specific neurological syndromes. In the clinical study, many intellectually retarded children and some children with other disorders (e.g., the hyperkinetic syndrome) showed overt neurological abnormalities of a kind that could not readily be classified under any of the headings provided on either the third axis or the ICD proper. These (quite common) non-specific neurological syndromes need codings.

A further problem concerned the principles underlying the third axis. Biological factors could be classified according to pathogenic influences, physical handicaps, or recognized medical conditions. The advantages and disadvantages of these approaches have been discussed by Tarjan et al. (*11*). It was decided to classify only medical conditions. Some participants felt that they lacked a means of coding some influences thought to be important in etiology. For example, there was no means of coding in accordance with the view that genetic factors were influential or that the disorder was due to low birth weight or perinatal damage. Whereas it was appreciated that polygenic hereditary influences might be important in the causation of child psychiatric disorders there was no means of determining their relative importance in individual cases. The same applied to perinatal factors. Accordingly, a coding could only reflect theoretical judgements, which, it was generally thought, should not form part of an international classification. It was also noted that a pathogenic approach had been followed in the fourth digit of the ICD mental retardation section and had proved to be highly unreliable.

Psychosocial factors

Most problems on the MAS arose with respect to the fourth axis, which concerned associated or etiological factors of a psychosocial nature, and it was concluded that this axis was unsatisfactory in its present form. First, there was disagreement on how psychosocial factors should be grouped. There were obvious unsatisfactory features in the scheme used in the present study but there was no consensus among the study participants on how it might be improved. It was recognized that much further research and discussion was needed before one could be achieved. Nevertheless, as psychosocial factors are such a crucial element in psychiatric diagnosis there should be further research in order to produce a better means of classifying them.

The second problem arose from the need to code several psychosocial factors. There was no logical reason why only one factor should be present, and in practice it was found to be common for several to co-exist. In these circumstances it is essential to have some instructions on how to decide which should have priority in coding and on how many codings to make.

The third problem concerns the question of severity. Most psychosocial variables are distributed on a continuum and it is therefore necessary to decide how severe a factor has to be before it can be coded. It is not meaningful to ask whether or not there is, for example, "social deprivation". Rather, one has to ask *how much* deprivation had occurred and code on the basis of the answer to that question. However, this necessitates instructions on how to grade severity and on how to decide what severity is required for a coding to be made. Such guidance was not provided in the study, but any acceptable scheme would have to include precise instructions on severity. Further research is needed before such instructions can be given.

Personality disorder

Personality disorder was diagnosed relatively infrequently and it was generally considered by participants that there were very considerable difficulties in diagnosing personality disorder in individuals still at an early stage of development. Nevertheless, the view was widely expressed that where the diagnosis could be made it was not logical to consider it as an *alternative* to acute psychiatric syndromes. Individuals could have an acute disorder (such as depression) in the context of a normal personality or against the background of long-standing personality disorder. The question of whether the personality was or was not abnormal was on a different dimension from that of the diagnosis of the acute clinical psychiatric syndrome. If this argument is accepted, the solution seems to be to put the question of personality on a different axis from that concerned with the clinical psychiatric syndrome. This approach is one frequently used in research but it would require a radical change in the style of clinical classification employed. This is not a matter that specifically concerns child psychiatrists but it is suggested that it would be valuable to investigate the possibility of classifying personality features or personality disorders as a separate axis.

Developmental disorders

Difficulties arose in the study because developmental disorders could be classified on either the first or third axis. This was found to be an unsuitable arrangement. There are considerable disadvantages in including developmental disorders with medical conditions as only a few have an unequivocal organic basis. On the other hand, there are difficulties in placing such disorders on a psychiatric syndrome axis because they so frequently co-exist with emotional or conduct disorders (*20, 21, 23*). It is suggested that in future studies of multiaxial systems of classifying child psychiatric disorder, developmental disorder should constitute a separate axis, on a trial basis.

Clinical psychiatric syndromes

A variety of problems arose with respect to the codings on the first axis. These are considered below in the discussion of child psychiatric disorders and the ICD.

Child psychiatric disorders and the ICD

The study findings clearly indicate the need for revision of section V when the Ninth Revision of the ICD is prepared if child psychiatric disorders are to be taken into account in the future. Four main issues emerged: (1) lack of codings, (2) lack of differentiation, (3) misleading groupings, and (4) combination categories.

Lack of codings

There are a few important disorders for which no specific coding is provided. The most important of these is "infantile autism", which at present is grouped under 295.8 with atypical forms of schizophrenia and schizophreniform psychosis. With such an arrangement it is not possible to identify infantile autism from among this heterogeneous group of disorders. The same applies to "anorexia nervosa", which is grouped with various feeding disturbances under 306.5, to the "hyperkinetic syndrome", which is included in the all-embracing 308 coding of "behaviour disorders of childhood", and to the "developmental speech disorders", which are lost in the 306.9 category of "other special symptoms not elsewhere classified".

Lack of differentiation

The majority of child psychiatric disorders (58% in this study) were lumped together under 308 (behaviour disorders of childhood). This is a most unsatisfactory category because it fails to differentiate among disorders that are unalike in symptomatology, pathogenesis, and outcome. It is also unsatisfactory because the inclusion terms list items such as "masturbation", which most child psychiatrists would regard as normal and of no psychiatric significance. Coding 307 (transient situation disturbance), as used for adults, also fails to distinguish between different types of disturbance, so that Ganser's syndrome, combat fatigue, and adolescent situational reaction are all grouped together.

Misleading groupings

In so far as "infantile autism" can be coded, it is included under schizophrenia (295). Whereas this coding was once in accordance with clinical practice, it is no longer so in view of the evidence that schizophrenia and infantile autism are quite separate conditions (23, 24). Coding 306 (special symptoms not elsewhere listed) includes a mixture of relatively well-defined disorders that should be grouped elsewhere and a heterogeneous assortment of special symptoms. The defined disorders (such as specific developmental speech disorders and specific reading retardation) should be classified separately. At the third seminar in the WHO programme it was argued that disorders should not be classified separately on the grounds of age alone (9). This seems a sensible ruling but it is contravened by having the adjustment reaction of adolescence in one coding (307) and the adjustment reaction of childhood in another (308). Category 305 (physical disorders of presumably psychogenic origin) is an assortment of disorders, many of which can also be coded under other sections of the ICD. For example, hysterical paralysis of a leg may be coded under 305.1 (musculo-skeletal neurosis) or 300.1 (hysterical neurosis).

Combination categories

ICD-8 classifies physical disorders associated with mental retardation in a most unsatisfactory manner by means of a fourth digit coding, and a different means needs to be found to deal with this situation. Although the issue arises most often with mental retardation, the problem is in fact a more general one—namely, what provision to make and what instructions to give for when a psychiatric disorder of some kind is associated with a physical condition.

Specific suggestions are made below as to how these difficulties might be resolved within the confines of the present structure of the ICD.[a]

---

[a] When this study was being carried out, the ICD-8 was in operation. As noted earlier, that edition was planned at a time when child psychiatric knowledge was more limited than it is now, and before systematic studies of classification had been undertaken. Accordingly, the limitations in ICD-8 that were evident in the present investigation reflect the inadequacies of psychiatry over a decade ago rather than any drawbacks in the ICD as such. It was for this reason that WHO established a programme of research (of which this study was one small part) to provide the knowledge needed for the next revision of the ICD. Partly as a result of that research programme, section V of the ICD is being revised for ICD-9. At the time of writing, proposals for ICD-9 have been made that meet most of the points raised in this report. However, the discussion of suggestions has been retained in order to illustrate how research findings may be used to promote improvements in classification.

Suggested revision of the ICD to include child psychiatric disorders

Psychoses

There are a number of psychotic conditions that always begin in childhood and are not provided for in ICD-8. A new 3-digit category is needed for these. There are two major conditions, infantile autism and disintegrative psychosis, that should be included here, but provision is also required for the variety of atypical psychoses specific to childhood (*23*). This new category should exclude psychotic disorders of a type that may begin in childhood but more usually start in adolescence or adult life. Thus, schizophrenia beginning in childhood would be coded under 295 as it is at present, manic-depressive psychosis under 296 as now, and organic psychoses under whatever codings are provided for these conditions in adults.

The −.0 coding in the new 3-digit category for "psychoses beginning only before puberty" could be used for "infantile autism" (or Kanner's syndrome), defined as a disorder beginning before the age of 30 months and characterized by an autistic-type failure to develop interpersonal relationships *and* a delay in language development *and* ritualistic or compulsive phenomena (*25*). This category should be used irrespective of evidence of organic brain pathology. Where a neurological disorder is associated with autism the neurological disorder should be coded separately.

The −.1 coding could be used for "disintegrative psychosis" (or Heller's syndrome), defined as a disorder in which normal or near-normal development for the first $2\frac{1}{2}$ years is followed by a loss of social skills and of speech together with a severe disorder of emotions, behaviour, and relationships. Again, where there is an associated neurological disorder this should be coded separately.

The −.8 coding could be used for "other" psychoses beginning only before puberty. This would mainly apply to the variety of atypical psychotic disorders that may be found in mentally retarded children.

The −.9 coding could remain for unspecified types of child psychosis.

The suggested scheme is shown in Table 25.

TABLE 25
PSYCHOSES WITH AN ORIGIN SPECIFIC TO CHILDHOOD

	.0	Infantile autism
	.1	Disintegrative psychosis
	.8	Other
	.9	Unspecified
Schizophrenia		classify as for adults
Manic-depressive psychosis		classify as for adults
Organic psychoses		classify as for adults

Specific delays in development

In the ICD-8, disorders involving a specific delay in development are grouped together under coding 306 with a heterogeneous mixture of special symptoms and disorders, a most undesirable arrangement, since the disorders with developmental delay have a conceptual unity and also there is substantial empirical evidence linking them as group and separating them from other conditions. The specific delays all concern skills that are related to biological maturation, a delay in one skill is often associated with lesser delays in other skills, there is a characteristic and similar age trend in all disorders (improvement with increasing age), and the disorders all show a very marked preponderance in boys. The concept of a specific developmental disorder different from general intellectual retardation is supported by evidence from research (20).

The fourth digit for this category could be used to indicate which skill is delayed in development, according to a scheme along the lines of Table 26.

TABLE 26
SPECIFIC DELAYS IN DEVELOPMENT

.0	Specific reading retardation
.1	Specific arithmetical retardation
.2	Other specific learning difficulties
.3	Developmental speech/language disorder
.4	Specific motor retardation
.5	Mixed developmental disorder
.8	Other
.9	Unspecified

The scheme omits enuresis and encopresis, which might well have been included with specific delays in development. The reasons for exclusion are that (1) there is less overlap between enuresis/encopresis and the other specific delays than there is between the delays listed under that heading; (2) both enuresis and encopresis, unlike the other conditions listed, often begin *after* control has been acquired; and (3) both enuresis and encopresis appear to be less unitary disorders than the others listed, although none is a single disease entity (26, 21). In view of their differences it seemed preferable to retain enuresis and encopresis under "special symptoms not elsewhere listed", so that the 3-digit heading of "specific delays in development" should have greater meaning and greater homogeneity.

Mental retardation

For reasons already discussed, it is necessary to abandon the fourth digit pathogenic classification used for mental retardation in ICD-8. Instead, there should be instructions specifying that where there is an associated or underlying medical condition this should be coded separately under the appropriate category outside section V. With this change, it would be possible to cover mental retardation in one 3-digit category, using the fourth digit to specify severity. This would have the advantage of freeing some categories to provide for child psychiatric disorders. Alternatively, in view of the major pathological and educational differences between mild retardation and moderate or severe retardation (*19*), mild retardation could be given a separate 3-digit category. The only other change advisable would be to omit the "borderline mental retardation" coding, as suggested both by the WHO Expert Committee (27) and the fifth seminar in the WHO programme (*11*).

Certain practical points arose in the study with respect to rating the severity of intellectual impairment, and attention to these would be required in drafting the glossary. First, in order to avoid differences in coding arising from theoretical differences, the coding should be based on the child's level of intellectual functioning *without regard to its nature* (such as psychosis, cultural deprivation, mongolism, etc.). Secondly, the level should be based on the *current* level of functioning (so that a dementing child should be coded according to his present level, not according to his level prior to the dementia). Thirdly, where there is a marked difference between different aspects of cognitive functioning due to specific handicaps, the coding should be based on assessments of cognition *outside the area of specific handicap*. Thus, ordinarily, the intellectual level of a deaf child or a child with a specific developmental language disorder should be based on *non*-language tests, whereas the intellectual level of a blind child or a child with a specific visual perceptual handicap should be based on language tests. Fourthly, the assessment of intellectual level should be based on whatever information is available, including both clinical evidence and psychometric findings. In most circumstances an IQ score is the best single indicator of intellectual level but the score should not be applied rigidly and unthinkingly to produce a coding.

Disturbance of emotions specific to childhood and adolescence

In the past, the bulk of child psychiatric disorders have fallen into the general category of 308 (behaviour disorders of childhood). This vague and non-specific category no longer does justice to the state of knowledge in child psychiatry and further differentiation is obviously required. The major subdivision of the common child psychiatric disorders is between emotional or neurotic disorders on the one hand and conduct disorders characterized by socially disproved behaviour on the other. These two major groups differ in terms of symptom clustering, sex distribution, response to treatment, long-term prognosis, association with family discord, and scholastic difficulties (*16, 18*). Because they differ so fundamentally they must be given different 3-digit headings.

Traditionally, the disorders involving anxiety, misery, fears, obsessions, and the like have been called "neurotic" disorders. The question therefore arises why they cannot simply be coded under the category 300 used for adult neuroses. One reason is that many emotional disorders in childhood are relatively undifferentiated and do not fall readily into any of the recognized categories of adult neurosis. Perhaps a more important reason is that, in spite of surface similarities, the emotional disorders of childhood have surprisingly little continuity with adult neuroses (*23*). The sex distribution is not the same, most "neurotic" children do not become neurotic adults, and many neurotic adults do not develop their disorders until adult life. For these reasons it seems desirable to have a separate category for the conditions of childhood. For the same reasons it appears preferable to use a descriptive term such as "emotional disorder" rather than the word neurosis, which for some psychiatrists has etiological implications.

The next issue is whether all emotional disorders in childhood should be classified separately or whether some should be coded under adult neurosis. Present knowledge does not permit the differentiation of emotional disorders that are precursors of adult neurosis from those that are not. Nevertheless, to differentiate solely on age seems unsatisfactory. As a result, it is suggested that where the emotional disorder falls into one of the traditional categories of adult neurosis (as it often does, particularly in adolescents) it should be coded under 300. The coding of "disturbance of emotions specific to childhood and adolescence" should be restricted to the less well differentiated (and often milder) emotional disorders more characteristic of the childhood period.

The subdivision of emotional disorders poses further difficulties in view of the weak differentiation between different types of emotional disorder and because of the lack of a well-developed scheme. The American Psychiatric Association's diagnostic and statistical manual (28) makes the distinction between an "over-anxious" reaction and a "withdrawing" reaction. Study participants suggested that a category for relationship problems was also desirable. In addition, it was suggested that a category for misery and unhappiness would be appropriate as, particularly in young children, this problem often does not have the characteristics of depression as seen in adult life. Some child psychiatrists would like a category for "school refusal", but as this is a heterogeneous category that may arise on several different bases, and as school refusal may be due to depressive states or phobic reactions that already have a coding, it would be illogical to provide a separate overlapping category.

The scheme shown in Table 27 is therefore suggested; it should be recognized that the subdivisions are less well established than those in some other 3-digit categories but, in spite of this, subdivision is probably worth attempting.

TABLE 27
DISTURBANCE OF EMOTIONS[a] SPECIFIC TO CHILDHOOD AND ADOLESCENCE

.0	With anxiety and fearfulness
.1	With misery and unhappiness
.2	With sensitivity, shyness, and social withdrawal
.3	Relationship problems
.8	Other or mixed
.9	Unspecified

[a] Where emotional disorder takes the form of a neurosis described udner 300, the appropriate 300 coding should be used.

Disturbance of conduct in childhood

Conduct disturbances form the other large group of child psychiatric disorders and there was general agreement among the study participants on the need for such a category as provided in the MAS. Nevertheless, some participants were reluctant to use the category "conduct disorder" when there was no delinquency (although the glossary was explicit that it should not be confined to delinquent disorders). It was felt that the more general "disturbance of conduct" did not have this connotation and that the non-delinquent varieties of disturbance should be recognized by means of subdivisions of the disturbances of conduct category. There is no generally agreed subclassification of disturbances of conduct although a variety of schemes have been proposed (*29*). The most commonly recognized distinction is between "unsocialized aggression" and "socialized delinquency" (*30*) or between aggression and antisocial behaviour (*31*). The "aggressive" category seems generally satisfactory and should be used where quarrelling, fighting, disobedience, aggression, destructiveness, and temper tantrums constitute the main problem. The category of "socialized delinquency", in which the individuals share the values of a delinquent sub-culture, is more open to dispute as the items said to characterize this disorder have not always been found grouped together (*32, 18*). Nevertheless, in view of its wide usage—e.g., in the American Psychiatric Association's manual (*28*)—it is probably worth retaining.

One of the clear findings of the present study is the frequent occurrence of disorders in which disturbances of conduct and of the emotions co-exist. This is in keeping with the findings of previous studies using a different methodology (*18, 31*). It was generally agreed by the study participants that there should be a category for a mixed disturbance. Findings from this and other investigations are contradictory on whether such a mixed group has more in common with the "pure" disturbances of emotions or the "pure" disturbances of conduct, but on balance it seemed most appropriately placed here.

How far other subdivisions are needed is uncertain. The American Psychiatric Association's manual (*28*) lists the "runaway reaction" as a separate subdivision but this arrangement has been criticized (*33*) and study participants were doubtful whether it should be retained.

Some participants thought that there should be a separate category for sexual misconduct as this is a frequent problem among adolescent girls referred to psychiatrists. However, this category does not seem to have any conceptual unity and, as the American Psychiatric Association's manual notes, where such behaviour is abnormal it may be classified under "socialized delinquency".

Accordingly, the scheme shown in Table 28 is suggested.

TABLE 28
DISTURBANCE OF CONDUCT

.0	Unsocialized disturbance of conduct
.1	Socialized disturbance of conduct
.2	Mixed disturbance of conduct and emotions
.8	Other disturbance of conduct
.9	Unspecified

The "hyperkinetic" syndrome

The inclusion of a coding for the "hyperkinetic" syndrome was generally thought to be useful. However, there are problems with both its naming and its definition. Hyperkinesis is usually included in the name of the disorder but it is known that the overactivity seen in early childhood frequently diminishes with increasing age and may be replaced by underactivity in adolescence (*34*). Accordingly, it seems necessary that overactivity should not constitute an essential part of the definition. The features of short attention span and distractibility appear less age-specific and some participants thought that these might ultimately prove to be the central features of the condition. Nevertheless, it seemed undesirable at this stage to change the name of the disorder. To take account of the variation in the clinical manifestations of the disorder it was suggested that there should be a subdivision into an "overactive" type and an "other" type.

The question of what other conditions should be grouped together with the hyperkinetic syndrome allows of no easy answer. Many children with the disorder have speech, language, motor, and perceptual problems of a developmental type and, particularly in view of the similar sex distribution, it could be argued that the hyperkinetic syndrome should be placed with the developmental disorders. On the other hand, in a substantial minority of children the disorder is associated with organic brain pathology and for this reason it might seem preferable to classify it with the non-psychotic organic brain syndromes. However, developmental delays and organic brain pathology do not occur in many hyperkinetic children and for this reason both these alternatives seemed unacceptable. Another possibility would be to place the condition with the disturbances of conduct, as such disturbances are frequent accompaniments of hyperkinesis. But this combination, too, is far from universal and in view of the associated developmental and organic factors found in many hyperkinetic children it seemed sufficiently different from the other disturbances of conduct not to be put there. Another solution would be to divide hyperkinetic disorders into those due and those not due to organic brain pathology. However, this is not a distinction that can be made reliably and it remains uncertain how far the "organic" and "other" varieties of the hyperkinetic disorder differ in terms of clinical course and response to treatment. For all these reasons, it seemed best simply to place the hyperkinetic disorder in a 3-digit category of its own.

In order to take account of the varied clinical manifestation of the syndrome a fourth digit subdivision along the lines of Table 29 might be used.

TABLE 29
"HYPERKINETIC" SYNDROME OF CHILDHOOD

.0	Simple disturbance of activity or attention
.1	Hyperkinesis with developmental delay
.2	Hyperkinetic conduct disorder
.8	Other—specified
.9	Unspecified

Personality disorder

There are major conceptual and practical problems in diagnosing personality disorder in the child who has not yet reached maturity. However, in so far as personality disorder can be diagnosed in the child, there seems to be no good reason why it should be classified in a different way from that used for adults. Study participants were dissatisfied with the ICD subclassification of personality disorders but it was considered undesirable for child psychiatrists to develop a separate scheme, and whatever classification is used for adults should also be used for children.

Drug dependence

The ICD classification of drug dependence is equally appropriate for children as for adults. However, in all age groups there is the problem of how to classify disorders involving abuse of drugs that does not amount to dependence. A separate 3-digit category for these disorders would be useful.

Sexual deviations

The ICD-8 provision for the coding of sexual deviations gives rise to a difficulty for child psychiatrists in that, although disorders in adolescents may reasonably be classified as in adults (as shown by the case in the reliability study), there is no adequate provision for psychosexual disorders (such as feminism or cross-dressing in boys) occurring in sexually immature children. A fourth digit coding for these disorders would be useful.

Physical disorders of presumably psychogenic origin

The study included very few cases of physical disorder of presumably psychogenic origin. The grouping and definition of disorders in this 3-digit category is unsatisfactory but there is no reason why such disorders should be dealt with differently in the child. Some suggestions for modification have already been made during the discussion of multi-axial systems.

Adaptation reaction/transient situational disturbance

The study findings showed that the category of adaptation reaction, as used for generally mild disorders of good prognosis, was useful. However, it appeared unsatisfactory not to have a subclassification according to the type of symptomatology (as in other categories) and it is undesirable for the coding to be restricted to any one age group. It is suggested that it could be merged with the existing category of transient situational disturbance, as defined in the American Psychiatric Association's manual (28), and extended to all age groups. A scheme such as that shown in Table 30 might be appropriate.

TABLE 30
ADAPTATION REACTION/TRANSIENT SITUATIONAL DISTURBANCE

.0	Depressive reaction
.1	Predominant disturbance of other emotions
.2	Predominant disturbance of conduct
.3	Mixed disturbance of emotions and conduct
.8	Other
.9	Unspecified

Special symptoms or disorders not elsewhere classified

In any classification there is always a need for "special symptoms or disorders not classifiable elsewhere" and this applies to child disorders as much as it does to adult disorders. Provided the ICD scheme is modified by placing certain items elsewhere (as suggested above) there seems no reason why the same scheme should not apply to all age groups. However, certain modifications to the ICD-8 scheme are needed for all ages. First, the title should be expanded to include "disorders" as well as "symptoms", to cover conditions such as "anorexia nervosa" that are more than a special symptom. As discussed already, the distinctiveness of "anorexia nervosa" merits its being given a separate fourth digit coding. At present, for reasons which are totally obscure, Gilles de la Tourette's syndrome is coded 347.9 together with hydrocephalus, kuru, cerebellar ataxia, and other diseases of the brain. Clearly, it does not belong there. The available evidence suggests that the distinction between this syndrome and other disorders involving tics is not as clear-cut as was once thought (*35*). It is suggested, therefore, that tics and Gilles de la Tourette's syndrome be grouped together. A frequent problem in mentally retarded individuals in institutions is stereotyped repetitive movements. At present there is no obvious way in which these can be classified. It is suggested that a separate coding be provided. Accordingly, the scheme shown in Table 31 is suggested.

TABLE 31
SPECIAL SYMPTOMS/DISORDERS NOT ELSEWHERE CLASSIFIED

.0	Stammering/stuttering
.1	Anorexia nervosa
.2	Tics
.3	Stereotyped repetitive movements
.4	Specific disorders of sleep
.5	Specific disorders of eating
.6	Enuresis
.7	Encopresis
.8	Psychalgia
.9	Other or unspecified

The need for further research

The suggestions made above derive from our studies and from the relevant findings in the literature. The categories proposed should be workable but they require testing and many problems remain to be solved before a satisfactory classification of child psychiatric disorders can be developed. In the absence of well-based knowledge, some of the suggested groupings have necessarily been based on arbitrary decisions. There are many topics that require substantial research if rational decisions about classification are to be taken on a scientific basis in the future. The outstanding questions include the following. In what ways do mixed emotional and conduct disorders relate to "pure" emotional and "pure" conduct disorders? What links are there between the emotional disorders of childhood and the neuroses of adult life? How should conduct disorders be subclassified? What is the validity of the concept of subcultural delinquency unassociated with personal psychopathology? How often does depression occur in the prepubertal child, how is it manifest, and how is it related to depressive disorder in the adult? What is the nosological status of the hyperkinetic syndrome? To what extent are biological factors associated with delayed maturation important in the pathogenesis of enuresis and of encopresis? How far are the specific delays in development due to homogeneous syndromes? How can disorders of personality be diagnosed in the preadolescent child and how should such disorders be subclassified?

Conclusions

1. It has been shown that a multi-axial system of classification (MAS) has important advantages over a multi-category system as normally used. Its superiority was most evident in its handling of disorders in which a psychiatric condition was associated with a physical illness or with intellectual retardation. In both instances the MAS gave more information more systematically and in a more comparable form than did ICD-8. A further advantage was the differentiation possible within the multi-axial system between the clinical psychiatric syndrome and its etiological influences. All psychiatrists found that this possibility made classification both easier and more uniform in view of the continuing dispute on theory and on causation.

2. The use of the MAS in a series of over 200 consecutive new cases seen in ordinary clinical practice provided valuable information that was not obtainable from the case-history exercise. Participants found the MAS easy to apply because it corresponded more closely to their usual clinical approach and it was preferred to ICD-8 (when used without a multi-axial framework) in both theory and practice. The information demands of the MAS were modest and it was found that sufficient data were available in routine outpatient practice to make codings on all four axes. The statistical presentation of data from the MAS proved to be quite straightforward, being easier and more reliable than with ICD-8. The coding of clinical psychiatric syndromes on the MAS was found to be reasonably reliable in most instances and the major categories used proved meaningful in that most of them were differentiated in terms of age and sex distribution, symptomatology, family background, associated intellectual retardation, and/or prognosis.

3. It appears that the advantages of a multi-axial system should apply as much to general psychiatry as they do to child psychiatry, although the axes used would not necessarily be the same. Research is needed to study the application of this approach to adult disorders. In extending the approach to adults, particular attention would need to be paid to the development of an axis to classify personality variables or personality disorders.

4. Psychiatrists were agreed upon the value of coding associated or etiological psychosocial factors, but the particular codings provided on the MAS were found to be both unreliable and non-discriminating. Much further research is needed to develop an acceptable and workable scheme of classifying psychosocial influences.

5. It was found possible to classify child psychiatric disorders reliably and meaningfully, but the ICD-8 makes no adequate provision for such classification, being inadequate because of lack of codings, lack of differentiation, misleading groupings, and unsatisfactory combination categories. To remedy the situation, special categories are needed for psychosis with an origin

specific to childhood, for specific delays in development, for disturbances of emotions specific to childhood and adolescence, for disturbances of conduct, for the "hyperkinetic" syndrome, for disorders of developing psychosexual identity, and for "adaptation reactions" (mild and transient disorders of good prognosis). Ways were suggested of introducing these changes into the ICD-9 without altering the basic structure of the classification.

6. Most of the major categories in the suggested scheme are supported by some empirical research but further research is needed to substantiate, modify, or refute their validity and, in particular, the fourth digit sub-divisions put forward. Classification schemes can no longer be based upon theoretical discussions; the clinical facts upon which schemes of classifications stand must be firmly established by sound research. The distinctions between categories must be based upon clinically meaningful differences, and the reliability and usefulness of any scheme of classification must be determined by systematic studies and by field trials. A useful but small beginning has been made on the classification of child psychiatric disorders, but much further research is required to test and to develop schemes of classification.

References

1. Knibbs, G. H. The international classification of diseases and causes of death and its revision. *Medical Journal of Australia,* **1**: 2–12 (1929)
2. United Kingdom, General Register Office. First annual report of the Registrar-General of England and Wales, London, Her Majesty's Stationery Office, 1839
3. World Health Organization. *Basic documents,* 18th ed., Geneva, 1974
4. Stengel, E. Classification of mental disorders. *Bulletin of the World Health Organization,* **21**: 601–663 (1959)
5. Lin, T. The epidemiological study of mental disorders. *WHO Chronicle,* **21**: 509–516 (1697)
6. Shepherd, M. et al. An experimental approach to psychiatric diagnosis: an international study. *Acta psychiatrica et neurologica Scandinavica,* **44**: suppl. 201 (1968)
7. Kanner, L. The thirty-third Maudsley Lecture: Trends in child psychiatry. *Journal of Mental Science,* **105**: 581 (1959)
8. WHO Technical Report Series, No. 185, 1960 (*Epidemiology of mental disorders*: eighth report of the WHO Expert Committee on Mental Health)
9. Rutter, M. et al. A tri-axial classification of mental disorders in childhood. *Journal of Child Psychology and Psychiatry and Allied Disciplines,* **10**: 41–61 (1969).
10. World Health Organization. *Manual of the international statistical classification of diseases, injuries, and causes of death,* 1965 revision, Geneva, 1967
11. Tarjan, M. D. et al. Classification and mental retardation: issues arising in the Fifth WHO Seminar on Psychiatric Diagnosis, Classification and Statistics. *American Journal of Psychiatry,* **128** (11, suppl.): 34 (1972)
12. Essen-Möller, E. Suggestions for further improvement of the international classification of mental disorders. *Psychological Medicine,* **1**: 308–311 (1971)
13. Wing, L. Observations on the psychiatric section of the International Classification of Diseases and the British Glossary of Mental Disorders. *Psychological Medicine,* **1**: 79–85 (1970)
14. Kendell, R. F. Psychiatric diagnoses and how they are made. *British Journal of Psychiatry,* **122**: 437–445 (1973)
15. Rutter, M. et al. Preliminary communication: an evaluation of the proposal for a multi-axial classification of child psychiatric disorders. *Psychological Medicine,* **3**(2): 244–250 (1973)
16. Rutter, M. Classification and categorization in child psychiatry. *Journal of Child Psychology and Psychiatry and Allied Disciplines,* **6**, 71–83 (1965)
17. United Kingdom, General Register Office. Studies on medical and population subjects, No. 22: a glossary of mental disorders, London, Her Majesty's Stationery Office, 1967
18. Rutter, M. et al. Education, health and behaviour, London, Longman, 1970
19. Rutter, M. Psychiatry. *In*: Wortis, J., ed. Mental retardation: an annual review, III, New York, Grune & Stratton, 1971

20. Rutter, M. & Yule, W. Specific reading retardation. *In*: Mann, L. & Saratino, D., ed. The first review of special education, Philadelphia, Buttonwood Farms, 1973

21. Kolvin, I. et al. Clinics in developmental medicine, No. 48/49: Bladder control and enuresis, London, Heinemann/S.I.M.P., 1973

22. Rutter, M. and Martin, J. A. M., ed. The child with delayed speech, London, Heinemann/S.I.M.P., 1972

23. Rutter, M. Childhood schizophrenia reconsidered. *Journal of Autism and Childhood Schizophrenia*, **2**: 315–337 (1972)

24. Kolvin, I. Psychoses in childhood—a comparative study. *In*: Rutter, M., ed. Autism: concepts, characteristics and treatment, London, Churchill Livingstone, 1971

25. Rutter, M. The description and classification of infantile autism. *In*: Churchill, D. W. et al., ed. Infantile autism, Springfield, IL, Thomas, 1971

26. Anthony, E. J. An experimental approach to the psychophathology of childhood: encopresis. *British Journal of Medical Psychology*, **30**: 146–175 (1957)

27. WHO Technical Report Series, No. 392, 1968 (*Organization of services for the mentally retarded*: fifteenth report of the WHO Expert Committee on Mental Health)

28. American Psychiatric Association. Diagnostic and statistical manual of mental disorders (D.S.M. II), Washington, DC, 1968

29. Scott, P. D. Delinquency. *In*: Howells, J. G., ed. Modern perspectives in child psychiatry, London, Oliver & Boyd, 1965

30. Hewitt, L. E. & Jenkins, R. L. Fundamental patterns of maladjustment: the dynamics of their origins, Michigan Child Guidance Institute, 1946

31. Wolff, S. Dimensions and clusters of symptoms in disturbed children. *British Journal of Psychiatry*, **118**: 421–427 (1971)

32. Field, E. A validation study of Hewitt and Jenkins' hypothesis, London, Her Majesty's Stationery Office, 1967

33. Fish, B. Problems of diagnosis and the definitions of comparable groups: a neglected issue in drug research with children. *American Journal of Psychiatry*, **125**: 900–908 (1969)

34. Werry, J. S. Developmental hyperactivity. *Pediatric Clinics of North America*, **15**: 581–599 (1968)

35. Corbett, J. A. et al. Tics and Gilles de la Tourette's syndrome: a follow-up study and critical review. *British Journal of Psychiatry*, **115**: 1229–1241 (1969)

36. Helmchen, H. Problems in the use and acceptance of an international glossary to ICD 8. *In*: de la Fuente, R. & Weisman, M. N., ed. *Proceedings of the Fifth World Congress of Psychiatry, Mexico City, 1971*, Amsterdam, Excerpta Medica.

The axes, categories, and codings of the proposed multi-axial classification of child psychiatric disorders

FIRST AXIS—CLINICAL PSYCHIATRIC SYNDROME

0.0 Normal variation
1.0 Adaptation reaction
2 Specific developmental disorder
    2.1 Hyperkinetic disorder
    2.2 Speech and language disorder
    2.3 Other specific learning disorder
    2.4 Abnormal clumsiness ("developmental dyspraxia")
    2.5 Enuresis (as isolated disorder)
    2.6 Encopresis (as isolated disorder)
    2.7 Tics
    2.8 Stuttering
3.0 Conduct disorder
4.0 **Neurotic** disorder
5 Psychosis
    5.1 Infantile
    5.2 Disintegrative
    5.3 Schizophrenia
    5.4 Other
6.0 Personality disorder
7.0 "Psychosomatic" disorder
8 Other Clinical syndrome
    8.1 Acute confusional state
    8.2 Dementia
    8.3 Gilles de la Tourette's syndrome
    8.4 Anorexia nervosa
    8.5 Any other clinical syndrome
9.0 Manifestation of mental subnormality only (but not including any of the listed syndromes)

SECOND AXIS—INTELLECTUAL LEVEL

0 Normal variation in intelligence
1 Mild retardation

2 Moderate retardation
3 Severe retardation
4 Profound retardation
5 Retardation: degree cannot be estimated
9 Totally unknown whether child is retarded or not

THIRD AXIS—BIOLOGICAL FACTORS

0 *Non-neurological conditions*
    0.0 No physical disorder (neurological or non-neurological)
    0.1 Infective and parasitic (000–136)
    0.2 Neoplastic (140–239)
    0.3 Endocrine, nutritional, and metabolic (240–279)
    0.4 Blood and blood-forming organs (280–289) and circulatory system (390–458)
    0.5 Respiratory system (460–519)
    0.6 Digestive system (520–577)
    0.7 Genito-urinary system and complications of pregnancy, etc. (580–678)
    0.8 Diseases of skin and subcutaneous tissue (680–709)
    0.9 Diseases of musculo-skeletal system and connective tissue (710–718)
    0.X Other non-neurological conditions
        (If any of the above conditions also involve the nervous system, they should NOT be coded here. Rather they should be coded under the appropriate neurological heading)
1 *Infections and post-infective immunological disease of central nervous system*
    1.0 Bacterial, spirochaetal, viral, or protozoal intra-uterine infection
    1.1 Bacterial meningoencephalitides (including tuberculous meningitis, etc.) (013–8; 030–9; 320–4)
    1.2 Cerebral abscess (322)
    1.3 Viral diseases of the central nervous system (040–079)
    1.4 Post-infective encephalopathies thought to be related to immunological reactions (e.g., post-exanthematous encephalopathy, post-vaccinial encephalopathy)
    1.5 Encephalopathies otherwise associated with infection (e.g., Sydenham's chorea, sub-acute inclusion body encephalitis) (392)
    1.6 Phlebitis and thrombophlebitis of intracranial venous sinuses (321.0)
    1.7 Other infections and post-infective immunological disease of central nervous system
2 *Neoplasms and vascular disease*
    2.0 Malignant neoplasms of brain (191)
    2.1 Secondary neoplasms affecting brain (196–9)
    2.2 Neoplasms of lymphatic and haematopoetic tissue affecting brain (200–207)
    2.3 Benign neoplasms of brain (225)
    2.4 Neoplasms of brain—unspecified (238)
    2.5 Other neoplasms
    2.6 Cerebro-vascular disease (non-infective, but including sub-arachnoid haemorrhage, cerebral haemorrhage, thrombosis, embolism, and aneurism) (430–438 and 442)

2.7 Migraine (346)

2.8 Syncope (435)

2.9 Other vascular disease affecting central nervous system

3 *Nutritional and metabolic abnormalities affecting central nervous system*

3.0 Congenital disorders of amino acid metabolism (270)

3.1 **Congenital abnormalities of carbohydrate metabolism (including muco-polysaccharidoses,** glycogen storage disease, spontaneous hypogly-caemias—e.g., leucine sensitivity, galactosaemia) (271)

3.2 Congenital abnormalities of lipid metabolism (including Tay-Sachs disease, Niemann Pick disease, Gaucher's disease, metachromatic and other leucodystrophies) (272)

3.3 Miscellaneous congenital disorders of metabolism (e.g., Wilson's disease, porphyria, idiopathic hypercalcaemia) (273)

3.4 Metabolic abnormalities of central nervous system secondary to endo-crine dysfunction (e.g., hypothyroidism, hypoparathyroidism, secondary hypoglycaemia) (240–246, 250–258)

3.5 Primary nutritional deficiency (260–269)

3.6 **Acute toxic encephalopathies (including lead poisoning, renal failure, hepatic** failure, hypoglycaemia)

3.7 Other

4 *Chromosomal abnormalities*

4.0 Trisomy 21

4.1 15/21 Translocation

4.2 21/22 Translocation

4.3 Autosomal chromosome deletion

4.4 Trisomy other than 21

4.5 XO

4.6 Additional X chromosome or chromosomes (XXY, XXXY, etc.)

4.7 Other abnormality of sex chromosomes (XYY, etc.)

4.8 Other chromosomal abnormality

5 *Congenital malformations of central nervous system not associated with gross chromosomal abnormalities*

5.0 Rubella or other infective embryopathies

5.1 Drug radiation or other toxic embryopathy

5.2 Congenital malformations of neural tissue (e.g., microcephaly, poren-cephaly, microgyria, Moebius syndrome) (743)

5.3 Malformations of ventricular system (e.g., hydrocephalus) (742)

5.4 Cranio-facial malformations, and malformations of the first branchial arch, e.g. craniostenosis; Treacher Collins syndrome, hypertelorism, cleft palate, aglossia) (741, 745, 746, 749)

5.5 Miscellaneous malformations involving the central nervous system and other systems (e.g., Marfan's syndrome, Cornelous de Lange syndrome, **Laurence-Moon-Biedl syndrome, arachnodactyly, pseudohypopara-thyroidism**)

5.6 Other

6 *Heredo-familial and degenerative disease of central nervous system* (*without* **demonstrable chromosomal or metabolic abnormalities**)

6.0 **Familial white matter disease (e.g., Schilder's disease, neuromyelitis** optica (333)

6.1 Hereditary disease of striato-pallidal system (e.g., Huntington's chorea) (331)

6.2 Hereditary disease involving fibre tracts, cerebellar apparatus, and motor nuclei of brain stem and spinal cord (e.g., the hereditary ataxias, cerebellar degenerations) (332)

6.3 Neuro-cutaneous syndromes (e.g., von Recklinghausen's disease, tuberous sclerosis; encephalotrigeminal angiomatosis, incontinentia pigmenti, ataxia telangectasia, albinism)

6.4 Hereditary neuromuscular disease (muscular dystrophy)

6.5 Hereditary diseases of the peripheral nerves

6.6 Other hereditary and familial disease of or involving the central nervous system

7 *Specific developmental disorders*

7.0 Speech and language disorder

7.1 Specific learning disorder

7.2 Developmental dyspraxia (abnormal clumsiness)

7.3 Enuresis

7.4 Encopresis

7.5 Tics

7.6 Stuttering

7.7 Other

8 *Chronic neurological syndromes not otherwise specified*

8.0 Cerebral palsy of congenital or perinatal origin (of any type)

8.1 Postnatal cerebral palsy (of any type)

8.2 Uncomplicated (idiopathic) epilepsy

8.3 Chronic encephalopathy of any nature (not otherwise specified)

8.4 Progressive cerebral atrophy of unknown etiology

8.5 Other chronic neurological syndrome not classifiable elsewhere

9 *Disorders of the special senses, spinal cord, and peripheral nerves*

9.0 Disease of the eye (190, 224, 370–378)

9.1 Blindness, not otherwise specified (379)

9.2 Disease of the ear (380–387)

9.3 Deafness, not otherwise specified (388–389)

9.4 Acute disease or disorder of the spinal cord

9.5 Sequelae of disease or disorder of the spinal cord

9.6 Acute disease or disorder of the cranial (excluding optic and acoustic) nerves (e.g., trigeminal neuralgia) and peripheral nervous system (350–358)

9.7 Sequelae of disease or disorder of the peripheral nervous system

9.8 Headache, not otherwise specified (791)

9.9 Other

FOURTH AXIS—ASSOCIATED OR ETIOLOGICAL PSYCHOSOCIAL INFLUENCES

0 Normal psychosocial situation

1 Disorder of intra-familial affective relationships (e.g., hostility, lack of warmth)

2 Excess of parental control (e.g., overprotection, over-restriction)
3 Deficiency of parental control
4 Social or material deprivation (e.g., poverty, overcrowding)
5 **Experiential deprivation (e.g., lack of parent–child interaction, deficiency** of normal experiences)
6 Other psychosocial disorder

Summary of 17 case histories

Case history 1: John, aged 13

Referred because of very severe tempers at home. *Problem*—John had always been an irritable infant who needed frequent pacifying. About age 3 years he had developed frequent temper tantrums and had become over-close and clinging to his mother. He was reluctant to separate from mother for the first few months after starting school but soon settled down. His behaviour at school had not presented problems since then. However, at home he continued to be a tense, irritable, easily provoked child. At the time of referral he would lose his temper almost daily. Tantrums would last up to 45 minutes, during which he would be grossly destructive, shriek loudly, bang his head against the wall, hurl abuse at his parents, and threaten them with physical violence. He seemed most relaxed when his parents were depressed. At times he would cling to his mother and would look for opportunities to be near her physically and to take sides with her against his father. He was generally insulting and abusive to his father and seemed jealous when his parents showed affection to each other. He was often tense and low-spirited for short periods. His appetite was poor and he had difficulty getting to sleep at night. He had few young friends. *Past history*—normal pregnancy and delivery, normal milestones, no separations, no educational difficulties. *Family history*—father passive, mild-mannered man who had difficulty showing his feelings. Mother suffered from frequent headaches, and brief spells of depression. Acquiescent character and had great difficulty disciplining John. Parents happily married with a close affectionate relationship. Housing was adequate and there were no financial difficulties. *Investigation*—IQ 119. *Follow-up*—until the age of 16 with little change being noted in his behaviour.

Case history 2: Harry, aged 13

Referred because of inability to walk. *Development of complaint*—normal behaviour before the age of 5. Between the age of 5 and 11 missed much schooling because of frequent attacks of abdominal pain. No physical cause for the pain ever found. He was a moody, determined boy who usually got his own way with his parents. At the age of 10 remained off school for 3 months following a trivial accident whilst running. He said he was unable to walk after this and finally recovered only after being offered a pet dog if he would start to walk again. One year before the current referral his mother had been admitted to hospital for a time, during which he was often alone at home during the day. Neighbours noted that he became very anxious and admitted to fears that the house would collapse on top of him. Ten months before his referral he developed a progressive weakness of one arm following a minor injury. This coincided with a period of open hostility between his parents, when they discussed separation. Eight months before referral he lost the use of his leg and was confined to bed. Mother gave up her job in order to look after him and both parents showed concern for him and quarrelled less between themselves. He became increasingly aggressive and irritable and refused to allow anyone to touch his affected limbs. *Personal history*—normal pregnancy and development, normal milestones, no separations, no scholastic difficulties. *Family history*—elderly mother who had a long history of trivial somatic complaints. She had received inpatient psychiatric treatment for depression. Very close to Harry and confided in him details of her husband's infidelities and her own unhappiness. Father—taciturn, morose, irritable man, frequently unfaithful to his wife, little contact with his wife or son during leisure time. Marriage had never been a happy one. *Social circumstances*—house in poor state of repair. No financial difficulties. *On investigation*—IQ 111, no scholastic difficulties, no physical abnormalities detected. *Follow-up*—admitted to hospital and walked unassisted within two days. After leaving school had unstable work career and was arrested for assaulting a policeman while drunk and for dangerous driving. Had a series of girl friends but formed no stable relationships.

Case history 3: Andrew, aged 6, eldest of two siblings

Referred because of a fear of dogs. *Development of complaint*—he started to develop a fear of dogs at the age of a year, when the family lived next door to a garden in which there were two noisy hounds. These dogs never attacked Andrew and never came into the family's house or garden. Fear of dogs persisted after the family changed home and left the neighbourhood. At the time of referral he would run out into the middle of the road regardless of traffic if he saw an unleashed dog in the street. He would sometimes refuse to go shopping or visiting with his mother or go to the beach lest he should meet a dog. He would become anxious if he saw a film with a dog in it and would then bite his nails. Mother had tried to get him used to dogs by buying him a small puppy but he had been very anxious when this was done. He had no other fears and was not made anxious by any other animal. He was usually a happy boy and there were no other behaviour problems at school. At school he was bright and did well at his lessons. He had very few friends of his own age. *Past history*—normal pregnancy, delivered by Caesarean section because of fetal distress, normal milestones. *Family history*—mother reliable, sensible person, affectionate but not over-solicitous. Father—office worker, rather bluff, outspoken man considered by his wife to be self-centered and inconsiderate, rarely played with the children and took no part in making domestic decisions. The couple had frequent rows over father's lack of involvement in home life and mother regarded the marriage as an unhappy one. *Social circumstances*—adequately housed, no financial difficulties. *Follow-up*—considerable improvement with desensitization treatment. A year after referral he had little, if any, social handicap although he still tended to avoid unleashed dogs encountered unexpectedly. He was noted to be often moody at home.

Case history 4: Thomas, aged 15

Referred because of cross-dressing. *Development of complaint*—at the age of 3 he used to enjoy walking with both his legs in one trouser leg. Started secretly to dress in women's clothing at the age of 11. This practice discovered four months before referral when found lying asleep in his mother's and sister's underwear. After this he continued to dress up secretly in the bathroom. He said that he enjoyed the touch of the clothes rather than their appearance and expressed no wish to go out in public dressed in women's clothing. He walked in an effeminate manner and had several effeminate gestures. He worked as a part-time hairdresser's assistant during the weekends. His twin sister was said to be more achieving and aggressive than him. He was generally meek and passive, rarely showing signs of anger and accepted punishment or teasing without complaint. He often said that his siblings were better at most things than he was although he boasted about his ability to play the flute and to walk cross-country. *Past history*—pregnancy complicated by severe toxaemia. Delivered at 37 weeks. Normal milestones. *Family history*—mother in her mid-thirties, lively, intelligent, cheerful, sociable woman, lifelong interest in amateur operatics. Dominant role in bringing up children and making decisions at home. Father same age, moody, undemonstrative man, high standards in his work, found difficulty in talking to his children and spent little leisure time with them. Marriage had mostly been happy but more recently the couple had been growing apart and mother was currently concerned that father might be unfaithful. *Social circumstances*—adequate housing, no financial difficulties. *Investigations*—normal intelligence, normal genitalia, facial hair and acne present but no pubic hair. Voice high-pitched. IQ 100. *Follow-up*—a year after initial assessment denied cross-dressing but admitted to frequent desire to dress as a woman.

Case history 5: Kevin

Referred at the age of 13 because of social withdrawal, depressed mood, and academic underachievement. *Development of complaint*—Kevin was first thought to be a problem at the age of 5 when he started school. He had difficulty making friends, he was frequently tearful, and he refused to eat school dinners. Between the age of 9 and 11 he changed schools three times because of difficulties in "settling down". Made few friends and complained that other children picked on him and bullied him. Teachers confirmed that this was so but that Kevin never retaliated when teased or picked on. He often seemed unhappy and would become very anxious about homework, complaining that he found it difficult to concentrate. He worried if he could not complete his set work but always deferred doing homework until the last moment. He had been considered an intelligent boy and had been placed in a grammar school, but during the year before his referral his academic achievements fell off steadily.

At the time of his referral he was increasingly low-spirited, was having difficulty getting off to sleep, and frequently complained of abdominal pains and headaches, although his appetite was good. He had developed a mild mannerism at the age of 11 of rubbing his hands together and this had persisted and often led to his being teased. He was very close to his mother although he could lose temper with her. He got on poorly with his father, who, in turn, was intolerant of his sensitivity and his social difficulties at school. *Personal history*—normal pregnancy and delivery, normal milestones, separation from mother at age of 2 for 6 weeks whilst she was hospitalized for treatment of a complication of pregnancy. At that time he was unhappy and difficult to console. *Family history*—mother in middle thirties. She considered herself to be dominant in the marriage and was a rigid, anxious woman, subject to bouts of depression. She had a masculine appearance and wore manly dress. Father many years older than mother. He did night work. A placid, subdued man but quick-tempered and impatient with Kevin. He openly preferred Kevin's younger sister. *Investigations*—full-scale IQ, 120. His speech was slow with many long pauses between words. He appeared bewildered and somewhat vague. No hallucinations or delusions. Said he felt depressed and desperate about continuing at school and about his inability to communicate with either of his parents. He also described feeling apart from reality and said this made him feel very anxious. *Follow-up*—became less depressed after admission to hospital and treatment with amitriptyline but over the following 4 years had recurrent periods of depression associated with suicidal thoughts.

Case history 6: Paul

Referred at the age of 6 because of overactivity, poor concentration, and aggressive behaviour towards teachers and other children. *Development of complaint*—as an infant he would frequently scream and bang his head, and was restless and slept poorly. He was a noisy, irritable toddler who masturbated frequently, and mother found herself unable to cope with him. As a result she left Paul with a child-minder during the day while she went to work. The child-minder found him a very difficult child to control. At the age of 4 he was seen by a psychiatrist because of frequent screaming attacks, aggression towards other children, messiness, and an inability to play constructively with toys appropriate to his age. He was treated in a group of other disturbed children and became less overactive and aggressive. At the age of $4\frac{1}{2}$ he went to a nursery school but was excluded after 6 months because of his difficult behaviour. This pattern was repeated at two other schools, including one that specialized in difficult children. At the time of his referral his mother complained that he was always "on the go", that he showed unbridled aggression towards other children, masturbated incessantly, frequently attempted to undo men's trousers and women's blouses, soiled himself, and ate faeces and other inedible substances. He was clumsy and lacked any awareness of danger, enjoyed banging, screaming or screeching, often broke his own toys, and was cruel to animals. He lied and was disobedient. His relationship with his mother alternated between being very clinging and abusing and tormenting her. He often seemed unhappy and tearful, was afraid of thunder and loud noises, and was frequently incontinent of faeces. He slept poorly and woke early; he had a good appetite but was messy at the table. Previous treatment with chlorpromazine had not resulted in any improvement. *Past history*—pregnancy complicated by antepartum haemorrhage. No neonatal abnormalities. Did not sit until 9 months. Walked at 18 months. No recognizable words until the age of 3 and no simple sentences until the age of 4. *Family history*—father in mid-thirties, previously treated for depression. Happy-go-lucky, outgoing man, enraged by Paul's misconduct and responded by losing temper and striking him. Mother—younger than husband. Previously placid and good-natured but at time of referral depressed and irritable and preoccupied with her failure to control Paul's behaviour. *Investigations*—on examination, grossly overactive, little organized play. Speech difficult to understand—many omissions and mispronunciations. Clumsy and had difficulty with fine motor movements. EEG normal. Full-scale IQ 70, performance 58, verbal 87. *Follow-up*—gradual improvement over 4–5 years. When seen at the age of 14 he was still disinhibited and overactive, his speech remained jerky and indistinct, and his IQ was unchanged.

Case history 7: Kim

Referred at the age of 6 because of tearfulness and misery. *Development of disorder*—serious disharmony between mother and father during the first 12 months of Kim's life, culminating in separation. When Kim was aged 1 she went to live with her paternal grandmother and stayed with her until aged 4. During this time she saw her mother only infrequently. Sent for by mother at age 4 and immediately started to show signs of disturbance, which had not been present while she was living with her grandmother. She cried frequently for trivial reasons. She would cry when she wanted to use the lavatory, when she mislaid anything, or when she bumped herself accidentally. Also cried frequently when she was in class. Mother found Kim's crying made her anxious and responded to it by slapping her. If Kim was ignored she would usually stop crying spontaneously within a few minutes. She was generally an obedient and rather submissive child and enjoyed being near her mother. She had close friends at school. She slept well but would wake early. Appetite normal. Frequently asked to go to the toilet during the day. Her teachers considered her to be a squirmy, fidgety, overactive child who was occasionally miserable and unhappy, but in other respects they thought her to be normal and never noted that she was anxious or fearful. *Family history*—father was an intelligent man with a long criminal history. Had not lived with his wife or daughter for the past 5 years. Mother—anxious, tense woman of low average intelligence, living with a warm, concerned but happy-go-lucky and indecisive man, currently unemployed. Investigations—IQ 111, friendly cooperative manner, described feeling unhappy and missing her grandmother. Described dreams in which she was taken away from her mother by a large witch. *Follow-up*—responded well to maternal counselling and support and was considered to have made a complete recovery one year after her initial referral.

Case history 8: Lorraine

Referred at the age of 10 because of refusal to go to school, abdominal pains, dizziness, fears of the dark, and preoccupation with fears of death. *Development of complaint*—before starting school at 5 Lorraine had been an exceptionally clinging child, following her mother wherever she went. She started school without difficulty and seemed happy there. At the age of 6 her parents separated briefly but Lorraine showed no obvious concern. When she was 8 her father suffered from an abdominal emergency and there was open discussion in the family about how he nearly died. Lorraine showed no undue concern, nor did she a few months later when her grandmother was taken to hospital after a stroke. A few months later she was told off in class for talking and the following day refused to go to school and was tearful and anxious. The next day she returned to school and attended regularly for the rest of that term. However, she refused to return to school after the holidays. She cried, tried to hide, and complained of abdominal pain and dizziness. Mother tried repeatedly to take her to school but on each occasion she ran back home. The family practitioner suggested that she be allowed to stay home for a few days, and so long as there was no discussion about school she appeared well and happy. She remained off school and several weeks later started to sleep badly and said this was because she was lying awake fearing that she would die. She often spoke of her father's health and asked whether he would die. She expressed concern that her abdominal pain would lead to her death. Her previous academic performance had been average. Socially she was close to one very good friend and when not with her she seemed lost, discouraged, and unhappy. She was generally a placid, rather retiring girl who disliked competitive situations and was a poor loser. She was very close to her mother. Her mother felt that she was over-sensitive and commented that she would never tolerate contradiction or criticism. She bossed her younger brother and usually got her own way with her father. *Past history*—premature and forceps delivery, kept in an incubator for 7 days. Placid infant, normal milestones, continued to wet the bed until the age of 6. *Family history*—mother tense, anxious woman subject to periods of depression for which she had received psychiatric treatment. Admitted that she could never be firm with Lorraine. Father—self-employed, history of youthful delinquency. Quick-tempered man, frequently unfaithful to his wife, and inconsistent with discipline. *Social background*—poor housing, whole family shared single room, numerous and life-long acquaintances nearby. *Investigations*—IQ 111, no educational backwardness. Marked anxiety about separation from mother during examination. *Follow-up*—supportive treatment given and Lorraine returned rapidly to school. No further episodes of school refusal during two years of follow-up.

Case history 9: Barry, aged 14

Development of complaint—always a solitary child but at the age of 7 started to stay away from school and became disobedient and defiant. His class work deteriorated and he misbehaved at school. After the birth of his younger sibling, when he was aged 9, these behaviour disorders were exaggerated. He became increasingly aggressive, lost the few friends he had, and became unduly suspicious, accusing other children of looking at him and talking about him behind his back. At the age of 11 he developed various habits, including an insistence that he should eat food only with his own crockery and cutlery. When he used the toilet he demanded that his parents go into a particular room and shut the door. He had frequent temper tantrums during which he would scream, sob, roll on the floor, and then lock himself in his room. He invariably contradicted any expressed plans made by the family and he developed a number of facial tics and hand mannerisms and became very openly hostile to his father, abusing him, swearing at him, and occasionally hitting and accusing him of treating him unfairly. He was in frequent trouble at school and the other children thought him odd and were afraid of him. He disobeyed all the rules and frequently would walk around the classroom talking, apparently to himself. *Past history*—normal pregnancy and development, normal milestones. No serious illnesses or separations. *Family background*—father was an intelligent, articulate accountant. Known to be a litigious personality, repeatedly writing to his Member of Parliament and generally suspicious and hostile towards psychiatrists and school authorities involved with the family. *Mother*—younger than husband, thin, anxious, tearful woman. No overt marital problems, comfortably housed, no financial hardships. *Examination*—anxious, cold, remote child who felt that people were looking at him and talking about him. No evidence of any thought disorder or overt depression. No EEG abnormalities. Full scale IQ 95. *Follow-up*—complained about being discriminated against with great regularity at all clinic attendances, eventually ran away from home, and was placed in a boarding school where he was unhappy and got on poorly with all other pupils. At the age of 18 re-admitted to a psychiatric hospital because he was sure that people in the street were calling him names and commenting on his physical appearance; however, these ideas subsided within a few days of admission.

Case history 10: Penelope

Referred at the age of 7. *Complaint*—thought to be backward. As an infant she was unusually quiet, did not sit until the age of 11 months, and did not walk until 22 months. She had only 5 words in her vocabulary by the age of $3\frac{1}{2}$. She would frequently bang her head against the side of her cot. At the time of her referral she was attending a normal school but her speech was difficult to understand; she rarely spoke in front of strangers and frequently echoed. She was unable to cope with tasks and lessons set for her at school and could not read but could count up to 20. She was generally rather restless and was attentive only when watching television. She was affectionate towards her parents and enjoyed helping her mother with housework. However, she did not mix with other children and had no friends of her own age. *Past history*—normal pregnancy, no previous illnesses or separations. *Family history*—father was a teacher, no emotional or psychiatric problems. Mother—10 years younger than father, nervous, anxious woman. Two younger siblings developing normally. Marriage reported to be happy, housing adequate, no financial hardship. *Investigations*—no physical abnormalities noted, IQ 47, speech as reported above. *Follow-up*—at age 8 years excluded from ordinary school because of disruptive behaviour, home tuition for one year, and then placed at a special school. When seen at 14 years, her speech was much improved and she could carry on a conversation. Noctural enuresis had continued. There were daily temper tantrums; she was restless and fidgety and shy with strangers. Her social state had steadily improved but she continued to need supervision. Her IQ was 51.

Case history 11: Denise

Referred at the age of 8½ because of a marked deterioration in her behaviour during the previous 8 months. This was first noted by her schoolteacher, who thought that she was becoming increasingly vague and dreamy. At home she had become less interested in helping with the housework, seemed tired and listless, and was noted to walk into things. She was no longer able to do arithmetical calculation that had previously been within her grasp. She often stared into space. At times she would approach strangers indiscriminately and hug them or hang on to them. She seemed to have lost all sense of danger and wandered into the road, narrowly avoiding the traffic. Although previously able to play the piano she could no longer do so. Shortly before she was seen, she had lost the ability to eat with a knife and fork and had become incontinent of urine and faeces. Her speech was slurred and difficult to understand. *Past history*—normal pregnancy and development, measles at the age of a year, fell off a wall at the age of 7½ but did not lose consciousness. No fits at any time. Before the onset of her illness had been a lively, witty, outgoing child and had not posed any behaviour problems. *Family history*—no relevant physical or psychiatric illness. *Investigations*—on examination, mute, semi-stuporose child unable to recognize her parents, involuntary movements present in all limbs, associated with cogwheel rigidity. EEG showed repeated bursts of complex, high-voltage slow waves, CSF showed a first-zone rise. The patient died 8 days after admission and histological examination of the brain revealed changes compatible with subacute sclerosing leucoencephalitis.

Case history 12: Steven

Referred at the age of 8. *Complaint*—epileptic since the age of 3. Had recently become increasingly aggressive and restless. In addition to major convulsions he also had localized psycho-motor seizures during which he would be mute and needed feeding and taking to the toilet. These seizure states sometimes lasted for up to a week, and following the attack his speech would remain incomprehensible to strangers for several days and he would be unsteady on his feet and have no recollection of events that had taken place during the attack. These episodes occurred at approximately monthly intervals. Between attacks he was spiteful and aggressive to other children, disobedient and stubborn with his class teacher, unresponsive to disciplinary measures taken by his schoolteachers or his parents. He was disinhibited with strangers and would approach people in the street to ask them for money. Other children avoided him and he was teased and ignored by his siblings. He was unable to read. His memory for recent events seemed poor, although he often used to talk repeatedly about events that had happened many years before. He collected odd pieces of rubbish from the street and tried to give these to his father as a present or else would hoard them. He was exceptionally concerned with his own cleanliness, washed frequently, and would not wear clothes that were soiled in any way. He would insist on sitting in the same chair for each meal. At the time of his referral he was not receiving any anticonvulsants. *Past history*—no complications of pregnancy or delivery, normal milestones, no separations or serious illnesses. *Family background*—father was a rigid authoritarian person who worked as a shop assistant. Mother—easy going, rather untidy person who felt that she did not know how to handle Steven and was afraid lest she might do him any harm by reprimanding him. She feared that he would become insane and become a dangerous criminal. *On examination*—EEG revealed continuous bilaterally symmetrical 2-c.p.s. spike and wave activity. Normal skull X-ray and urinary chromatogram. Full-scale IQ 59. *Follow-up*—after control of his epileptic state he remained restless and disinhibited and continued to be aggressive and unpopular with other children.

Case history 13: Robert

Referred at the age of 9. *Problems*—he had not said his first word until the age of 4 and at the time of referral, despite lengthy speech therapy in the past, he still would only speak with people that he knew. When he spoke it was in a brief, telegraphic style indicating only his immediate needs. He echoed frequently and confused the sense of personal pronouns. He would be angry and anxious in unfamiliar surroundings and was upset if any of his toys or possessions were moved. He always insisted on sitting in the same chair. He often refused to eat solid foods but would drink large quantities of milk every day. He was very demanding and insistent and would push or pinch his parents or sister when contradicted or if not given his own way. He took no notice of people when they spoke to him and spent much of the day pacing up and down the room without apparent purpose or else totally absorbed in instructional games or jig-saw puzzles. He avoided eye-to-eye gaze. *Past history*—unwanted pregnancy, no complications. During early infancy was breast-fed for 9 months and mother felt very close to him. He was restless and it was difficult to get him to go to sleep. At the age of a year he started to rock in his cot and at the age of 18 months he started to bang his head. No separations until the age of 6. No formal schooling. *Family background*—father was an ebullient, extroverted, talkative man. Mother—15 years younger than father, generally depressed, withdrawn woman with many phobic and anxiety symptoms. She tended to be over-protective with Robert. *Investigations*—bilateral corneal capacities, jagged and sharp pointed teeth, no neurological abnormalities, positive blood and CSF WR. IQ—performance scale WISC 85, no verbal assessment possible, Vineland Social Quotient 47. *Follow-up*—diagnosis of congenital syphilis made. Treated with Penicillin. He retained numerous rituals but temper outbursts became less frequent in late teens. Apparently good at reading, but did so with little understanding. By age 18 spoke 2–4-word phrases, omitting all pronouns.

Case history 14: William, aged 13

Complaint—normal behaviour until the age of 11. At that time reported that he had been molested at the cinema by a man. He repeatedly referred to that incident, implying that he was now different from other boys. At the age of 12 he started to complain that other boys at school thought that he smelt and he spent hours on end in the toilet, using large quantities of lavatory paper. He stopped associating with other boys of his age but still spoke to younger children. He spent a lot of his time at home and in the class cringing in a corner and was often seen laughing to himself. He never left the house on his own and if either of his parents approached him he would run away to avoid them. He refused to let anyone, including his mother, touch the food he intended to eat; he cooked and prepared it himself. If by accident he touched one of his parents or sisters he would immediately go to the bathroom and wash himself. He always held his hand over his genitals and repeatedly plucked at his trousers. Sometimes he wore two pairs of trousers on top of each other and he would wear large numbers of clothes even on hot days. At night he was restless and complained of vivid nightmares. If any of his sisters' friends came to the house he would lock himself in the lavatory. He read a lot of comics and believed that the exploits recounted in them were real. *Past history*—normal pregnancy, development normal, never very forthcoming, always spoke less than his siblings. At the age of 2 he had a febrile convulsion. *Family history*—father was a heavy drinker. Mother—younger than father and had had a depressive illness in the past. *On examination*—detached, bizarre behaviour, laughing to himself without reason and muttering brief phrases. His talk was rambling and seemingly irrelevant and he repeatedly referred to having been sexually assaulted in the past. He was afraid that the doctor might kill him. He said that he always put his hand in front of his penis in case people should laugh at it. He admitted to hearing voices that accused him of being an idiot or daft and to hearing music. He thought that he had a spider in his head and that he deserved to be shot because an evil soldier's soul had entered his body. He attempted to mutilate his penis, saying that it was too big and filthy. *Follow-up*—there was no improvement with treatment and at age 22 years he was still an inpatient in a psychiatric hospital—dull, apathetic, noisy, impulsive, deluded, and hallucinated.

Case history 15: Claire

Referred at the age of $3\frac{1}{2}$ years. *Problem*—emotional upset, thought to be related to behaviour problems shown by her mentally retarded 5-year-old brother. She whined continuously, often had temper outbursts, and became increasingly clinging to her mother. She previously sat on the lavatory quite normally but now insisted on sitting on a pot. She had previously dressed herself but now demanded help in being dressed and fed. Parents related these changes to a deterioration in her mentally retarded elder brother's behaviour. The brother repeatedly tormented Claire and at times was dangerously violent with her. Both parents considered that as a result of the brother's behaviour they paid less attention to their other children. *Past history*—normal pregnancy and delivery, normal milestones, no serious illnesses or separations. *Family background*—mother was an intelligent, ambitious, talkative woman who fluctuated between being happy and optimistic and depressed and despondent. Father—modest, insightful, self-depreciating manner, calm and placid personality. Marriage was considered by both to be happy. Family financially comforable and well housed. *Investigations*—IQ 107. *Follow-up*—marked improvement in Claire's behaviour after her mother was treated with antidepressants and her brother had been placed in a special boarding school. She settled down well at school and made many friends. No problems when seen at the age of 6.

Case history 16: Gwen

Referred at the age of 11. *Main complaint*—incontinence of faeces since age 9. As an infant Gwen was characteristically constipated but was fully continent by the age of $2\frac{1}{2}$. At the age of 5 there was a brief period of faecal incontinence when Gwen started going to school, this lasted for approximately 2 weeks and at the time she complained that defaecation was painful. Soiling started again at the age of $8\frac{1}{2}$, when her elder sister left home. She soiled repeatedly throughout the day and also during the night. Her pants would be dirty within a few hours of a bath and soiling took place at school, at home, and when she was away on holiday. The faeces were always unformed. She only ever soiled her underwear and nightwear and sometimes hid the soiled clothing. She had some friends but was generally unhappy at school. At home she was usually cheerful and bossy and always keen to get her own way. There had been a single incident of stealing 3 years before but not since then. *Past history*—normal pregnancy and delivery, normal milestones. *Family background*—mother was an anxious woman who enjoyed work in an office. She felt guilty, thinking that working was in some way contributing towards Gwen's incontinence. Father—a fussy, tidy, meticulous person who was always nagging at Gwen to change her clothes and brush her nails and teeth. He regularly examined Gwen's clothing for signs of soiling and he supervised her bathing and generally treated her like a much younger child. The parents felt that their marriage was a close, sound, and happy one. Father stated that he felt closer to Gwen than to any of his other daughters. No social problems. *Examination*—faeces palpable per abdomen, no abnormality of rectal sensation, average IQ. *Follow-up*—treated with enemas and laxatives; faecal incontinence stopped and did not relapse.

Case history 17: Roy

Referred at the age of 14. *Problem*—referred for psychiatric opinion before appearing in court. As a young child he had a bad temper and stuttered but had no other disorders. He started to get into trouble at the age of 9 after his stepfather had been sent to prison. He was found stealing materials from a building site along with other boys. At the age of 11, after his stepfather had been released from prison, he was arrested for breaking and entering with another boy; two months later he was re-arrested on a similar charge. At the age of 12 he was arrested with a group of other boys attempting to break into a supermarket. At the age of 12½ he was seen by a psychiatrist, who recommended psychiatric treatment. However, this recommendation was resisted by the parents because they felt there was nothing mentally wrong with Roy. When on probation he visited his probation officer regularly and usually seemed cheerful. His attendance at school was good and he was always polite to the teachers and diligent at work. He enjoyed playing games and had many friends at school. He was fond of his family. Just prior to the present referral he had again been caught stealing with other boys who had a delinquent record. He was always concerned about his appearance, he ate and slept well, he never lost his temper and never appeared depressed. *Family history*—both his real father and his stepfather had a history of repeated convictions. His stepfather was an amiable, easy-going man who had a close relationship with Roy and often accompanied him on outings. Mother was described as a warm, loving woman, competent at handling her children but a poor manager with money. There were three younger half-siblings, none of whom had ever shown any disturbed behaviour. The family were currently well housed in local authority accommodation and were in receipt of social assistance. *Investigations*—IQ 109, no evidence of any acute mood or thought disorder.